Medical Pluralism

Medizin, Gesellschaft und Geschichte

Jahrbuch
des Instituts für Geschichte der Medizin
der Robert Bosch Stiftung

herausgegeben von
Robert Jütte

Beiheft 46

Medical Pluralism

Past – Present – Future

Edited by Robert Jütte

Franz Steiner Verlag Stuttgart
2013

Gedruckt mit freundlicher Unterstützung der Robert Bosch Stiftung GmbH

Umschlagabbildung: Der Ärztestreit. Kampf zwischen Homöopathie
und Allopathie. Relieffigur von Anton Sohn (1769-1841).
© Bildarchiv des Instituts für Geschichte der Medizin der Robert Bosch Stiftung

Bibliografische Information der Deutschen Nationalbibliothek:
Die Deutsche Nationalbibliothek verzeichnet diese Publikation in der Deutschen
Nationalbibliografie; detaillierte bibliografische Daten sind im Internet über
<http://dnb.d-nb.de> abrufbar.

© Franz Steiner Verlag, Stuttgart 2013
Druck: Laupp & Göbel GmbH, Nehren
Gedruckt auf säurefreiem, alterungsbeständigem Papier.
Printed in Germany
ISBN 978-3-515-10441-8

Contents

Preface

Robert Jütte

The recent widespread interest in alternative medicine points, in the words of Ted Kaptchuk and David Eisenberg, to a "dramatic reconfiguration of medical pluralism – from historical antagonism to what might arguably be described as a topical acknowledgment of postmodern medical diversity".[1] The question is, how the late 20th century birth of complementary and alternative medicine (CAM) resulted in yet another transformation in medical pluralism, locating quackery no longer in adhering to an unconventional treatment. The line of demarcation can now be found in a more ethical field, e.g. competency, qualifications, conduct, responsibility and personal professional development of a practitioner, almost regardless of the form of therapy in question. But does it really make sense to use the label "new pluralism"[2] coined by Cant and Sharma for this phenomenon?

These and other questions were addressed by a conference entitled "Medical Pluralism – Past and Present" which took place in the Villa Vigoni in Loveno di Menaggio (Italy) in May 2011. It was organized by the Institute for the History of Medicine of the Robert Bosch Foundation and the Centro Italo-Tedesco per l'Eccellenza Europea, in collaboration with the Dialogforum Pluralismus in der Medizin. Unlike previous conferences discussing medical pluralism in past and present[3], this symposium did not only focus on the tensions between orthodox medicine and other medical approaches within the cultural settings during the course of the 19th and 20th century. Any exploration of plural medicine including the historical perspective needs to be aware of the conflict between regular and irregular healers which existed already in the pre-modern era, although distinctive features such as "scientific", "alternative" or "traditional" which are so familiar to us today did not yet play a role. In the early modern period we observe a complex array of heterogeneous medical ideas and practices which has not much in common with the kind of pluralism or plurality which we can find in modern health care systems in Europe and non-western countries (e.g. India, Japan).

Comparing the medical market place in pre-modern, 19th, and early 20th-century Western Europe with the present situation in health care, the papers presented at this conference dealt with the historical development as well as with the present state of medical pluralism in and outside Europe. The papers selected for publication come up with data and evidence from a variety of sources, suggesting that unconventional medicine has been a persistent pres-

1   Kaptchuk/Eisenberg (2001), p. 189.
2   Cant/Sharma (1999), p. 194.
3   Cant/Sharma (1996); Gijswijt-Hofstra/Marland/Waardt (1997); Ernst (2002); Michl/Potthast/Wiesing (2008).

ence in health care over the past two to four hundred years. The contributors were drawn from different academic disciplines such as medical history, medicine, sociology, and anthropology. The chapters fall into two categories: those focused on forms of medical plurality in the age before the rise of biomedicine and those focused on medical pluralism today, bringing examples from Western European countries such as Italy, Germany, France, and Great Britain, but also from a country which has an outstanding reputation for practicing medical pluralism, India.

The contributors to this volume vary in the extent to which they engage with the theoretical perspective of the term medical pluralism, but each of them points out the underlying dynamics that had led to medical pluralism within different geographical and cultural settings and historical periods. Those chapters which deal with the medical plurality in pre-modern societies show that it was a long way before the tradition of healing became orthodox in the sense that a specific expert knowledge gained the logic and status to discredit other approaches as "quackery". They also explore the ideological and economic factors that contributed to the ways in which different medical systems were imagined as rational or irrational. If one fell ill in early modern times one had access to a considerable array of healers even if one was not well off. There were non-official or half-official specialists for all the more or less clearly defined afflictions: cutters of hernias, tooth pullers for toothaches, bone-setters (who usually also served as executioners) for dislocations, enchanters and wise women for lumbago. The case studies included in this volume (Gentilcore, Jütte, Ramsey) show that patients chose their healers horizontally or vertically, guided by aspects of reciprocity or the search for protection or, in other words, according to a social logic that they themselves determined. The term "medical pluralism" only applies with restrictions here. Prior to 1800, the healing system was neither homogeneous nor harmonious but riddled with conflict. We must nonetheless not base our description of these competing systems on the differentiations we make today between rational and irrational, natural and supernatural, religious and superstitious, especially when referring to the period prior to 1850 when this kind of dichotomy was still largely incomprehensible.

Those papers which focus on the 19th century (Marland, Nicholls, Baubérot, Stollberg) demonstrate that the process of professionalization that has penetrated the health care system since the 18th century had a lasting impact on the medical health care systems in England, France and Germany. The lay system – at least in theory – was no longer permitted to provide any medical services apart from nursing and care. Since the middle of the 19th century an increasing part of the population consulted medical experts when they were ill, even if they were not always university trained physicians but often semi-professional healers (e.g. non-academic surgeons and dentists). The social reasons for their behaviour are obvious. The degree of medicalization, or – more precisely – the density of physicians also played an important part in this. This change occurred as part of the overall modernization of society.

Today we have a clear dividing line between professional and other healers that is strictly monitored by the legislator, for the "benefit" of the patient. Non-medical practitioners nowadays have to undergo training and pass examinations before the relevant authorities to obtain a licence. Traditional healing rituals, reaching from faith healing to the charming of warts, although they survived, have been marginalised. The "new" pluralism requires that complementary therapists operate from a position of needing to establish their status as "experts". This means that the gap between CAM and conventional medicine may be much less than the general public believes, as the pressure exists that CAM should be judged by exactly the same standards used for conventional medicine (i.e. the rules established for an evidenced-based medicine).

The contributions collected in this volume tell us much about the ways in which diversity in medical health care has been achieved and practiced in different cultural and historical settings. They also tell us a lot about continuity and discontinuity, substantiating the findings by Cant and Sharma who stated: "The history of complementary medicine is discontinuous in that the emergence of a dominant medical orthodoxy pushed it into a particular position [...]."[4]

Bibliography

Cant, Sarah; Sharma, Ursula (eds.): Complementary and Alternative Medicines. Knowledge in Practice. London; New York 1996.

Cant, Sarah; Sharma, Ursula: A new medical Pluralism? Alternative medicine, doctors, patients and the state. London 1999.

Ernst, Waltraud (ed.): Plural Medicine, Tradition and Modernity, 1800–2000. London; New York 2002.

Gijswijt-Hofstra, Marijke; Marland, Hilary; Waardt, Hans de (eds.): Illness and Healing Alternatives in Western Europe. London; New York 1997.

Kaptchuk, Ted J.; Eisenberg, David M.: Varieties of Healing. 1: Medical Pluralism in the United States. In: Annals of Internal Medicine 135 (2001), no. 3, pp. 189–195.

Michl, Susanne; Potthast, Thomas; Wiesing, Urban (eds.): Pluralität in der Medizin. Werte – Methoden – Theorien. Munich 2008.

4   Cant/Sharma (1996), p. 20.

Medical Plurality, Medical Pluralism and Plural Medicine. A critical reappraisal of recent scholarship

Waltraud Ernst

Introduction

Since the 1980s and 1990s in the wake of debates on the role of Complementary and Alternative Medicine (CAM) within western societies, the term medical pluralism has flourished among historians and health policy makers in countries across the world. An appraisal of the continued currency of this concept and the insights garnered seems appropriate following nearly three decades of historical, anthropological and sociological studies of different historical and contemporary contexts. This will here be undertaken from the perspective of a social historian who has worked across disciplines, including cultural psychology, medical sociology and social history, with a particular focus on the social, political and cultural context of varied medical paradigms during the age of empire in Asia and the Pacific.

Existing work clearly attests to the fact that the field of healing in all periods and localities has been persistently characterised by a plurality of approaches, presenting a multitude of treatment options for patients in their pursuit of health. The extent to which developments in the late twentieth-century health care market in western countries have in fact been characterised by a "new" kind or a "dramatic reconfiguration" of medical pluralism has been widely debated.[1] Continuities between earlier and more recent periods are emphasised by some, and more current shifts in institutional authority in modern health care environments accentuated by others. Arguably, earlier concerns about the demarcation of "orthodox" versus "heterodox" approaches have been replaced more recently by a focus on the ethics and efficacy of practice regardless of the perceived conventionality of approach.

Two questions emerge. First, have the emergence of a "new pluralism" and the postulated shift from historical antagonism towards acceptance of medical diversity been substantiated? Second, has historical scholarship on medical plurality provided any new conceptual insights since its emergence a couple of decades ago; have there been new developments in the historiography of medical plurality? The first issue was to be investigated at the conference from which this essay results.[2] Here I will focus on the second set of issues, namely an assessment of the historiographic changes, if any, in the field

---

1   Cant/Sharma (1999); Kaptchuk/Eisenberg (2001).
2   Medical Pluralism – Past and Present. Organized by the Institute for the History of Medicine of the Robert Bosch Foundation, Stuttgart; Centro Italo-Tedesco Villa Vigoni, Loveno di Menaggio; in collaboration with the Dialogforum Pluralismus in der Medizin, Berlin (2011).

of the history of medical plurality. My reflections will mainly be based on the contributions presented at the conference to highlight some of the achievements in scholarship, the continued vibrancy of research and persisting gaps in the field.

"Viewing the Patient" versus "The Patient's View"

In his elegant contribution to "Patientenorientierung und Professionalität", Peter F. Matthiessen illustrated the plurality of medical paradigms and the varied cosmologies and ways of seeing and thinking going along with them by reference to Henry Moore's sculpture "Locking Piece".[3] Depending on the observer's perspectivity or angle of observation, the aesthetic appearance of the very same object varies considerably. Matthiessen is a medical practitioner and his aim was to highlight the scope for building bridges between followers of different medical paradigms, from the mainstream and the complementary medicine fields, by identifying their shared object of interest: the patient. It is in fact among the medical fraternity that the focus on the patient has been most significantly to the fore. "Patient-centred medicine" has during the last decade become a rallying call even for orthodox practitioners who had previously been criticised by patients and CAM healers alike for having lost touch with their main constituency since the heyday of modern, science-based medicine.

Intriguingly, among historians of medicine, patients and their families tend to figure less prominently in Anglo-American scholarship. This is despite the fact that earlier historical work on medical plurality was inspired by the paradigm of social history, which mooted a focus on the "view from below", namely the patients, rather than the traditional emphasis on medical policies and "big men, big ideas, and big institutions".[4] Admittedly, the continued, favoured choice of historical research perspective, which looks at medicine and sees varied medical concepts, a plurality of medical practitioners and a multitude of medical institutions and professional networks in the medical market place, has produced some path-breaking work. For example, heterodox and orthodox medical thought systems and practices and the roles, status and professional inclinations of their varied practitioners have been investigated in relation to different state policies in particular national and cultural settings – in western as well as non-western and post/colonial countries.

A recent example is the volume on "Medicine and the Market in England and its Colonies, c. 1450–1850", edited by Mark Jenner and Patrick Wallis.[5] It provides both geographically wide-ranging, in-depth case-studies of varied medical approaches and a cogent critique of the suitability of the concept of

---

3   Henry Moore, "Locking Piece". Bronze, 1963–64, Millbank, London. In: Matthiessen (2010), p. 99.
4   See, for the foundational statement on medical histories from below: Porter (1985).
5   Jenner/Wallis (2007).

the "medical marketplace" for pre-modern societies. Another example, in relation to non-western medical approaches, is Guy Attewell's path-breaking
"Refiguring Unani *tibb*. Plural Healing in Late-colonial India".[6] It focuses on
the varied ways in which a particular medical corpus was practised in late
nineteenth and early twentieth-century South Asia. Within the European context, historians working on the pre-modern period, such as Jütte, have deftly
employed anthropological methodology to explore healers' networks of practice and the complexity and fluidity of guilds.[7] However, in contrast to these
nuanced accounts of how the medical field is characterised by a plurality of
approaches and the recognition that practitioners are adaptable and versatile
in their approach to and vernacularization of codified and informal ways of
healing, patients and their families have remained neglected in historical research in the English-speaking world. Notable exceptions within the German
historiography include Dinges's work on patients in homoeopathy.[8]

A further problematical issue concerns the age-old challenge of "structure
and agency", which has plagued modern theorists from Durkheim to Bourdieu.
This is relevant in regard to historical as well as contemporary policy debates.
Even within frameworks that consider patients as active agents, as ever, the
structures within which this agency has been socialised and exerts its preferences still require attention. There is an ample literature in the field of the history of (post-)colonial medicine that explores this nexus particularly well. Any
investigation into medical plurality worth its salt is bound to investigate both
the legacy of structural constraints imposed by legal, religious and professional
authorities and particular interest groups and issues of resistance, subaltern
agency, continued pluralities, and emerging "multiple modernities" – in addition to an acknowledgment that patients and their families may have other
concerns than just the narrowly medical.[9]

In a similar vein, the best and most comprehensive medical anthropological research investigates the full spectrum of political, socio-economic and
personal parameters within which medical plurality manifests itself. Etsuko
and Eguchi for example explore patients' multiple realities and journeys
through varied treatment options available in modern Japan, ranging from
conventional medicine and hospital treatment to religious and shamanistic
practices.[10] Scheper-Hughes, perhaps more controversially, has highlighted
the role of the pharmaceutical industry in the medicalization of hunger and
starvation, exploring the social production of illness and patients' responses
within the constraints of the exploitative socio-political structures of north-east
Brazil and its flourishing medical market in her patient/structure-focused analysis of "The madness of hunger: Sickness, delirium, and human needs".[11] Such

6   Attewell (2007).
7   Jütte (1991).
8   Dinges (2002).
9   Ernst (2007).
10   Etsuko (1991); Eguchi (1991).
11   Scheper-Hughes (1988).

attempts by medical anthropologists to deal with medical plurality within more or less hegemonic and unabashedly exploitative socio-political and medical structures – while clearly putting the life-worlds and needs of patients, their families and communities at the centre of analysis – are still scarce in historical writing on medical plurality and medical pluralism in Europe.

A distinctive attribute of anthropological work has been its focus on patients to a far greater extent than historical research: on patients' and their families' varied perceptions of health and illness; on their diverse illness behaviours; and on their active role in seeking out particular practitioners and medical paradigms aligned with different medical systems (what has been called "healer hopping"). Arthur Kleinman has spearheaded this work and established a school of thought and research methodology that focuses on "illness narratives", namely sick people's narratives about their illnesses and the effect on their lives.[12] In contrast, the way in which the historians participating at the meeting at the Villa Vigoni interpreted their task of providing résumés of medical plurality in a number of western countries remained almost exclusively focused on particular groups of heterodox medical practitioners, their un/official treatments and professional networks, on the one hand, and state policies, professional regulations and, somewhat more testing, the role of self-help movements, on the other. Just one contribution foregrounded the agency of patients rather than the structures within which patients and their families are situated. But even here the investigation accentuated the media (domestic medicine books) to which patients referred for self-medication. For historians, so it seems, the term "medical pluralism" is still mainly perceived from and circumscribed by the perspective of medical discourse and treatments, the structures of professional organisation, state regulation and the networks of healers. The perspective by which the agency of patients and their families could be gleaned still remains largely unexplored. In contrast, for practitioners from complementary and, increasingly, orthodox medicine backgrounds, the patient has moved to the centre of analysis.

Framing the Patient

Practitioners of all stripes in Europe and North America have become acutely aware of the fact that there ain't no medicine and no doctor – qualified in conventional medicine, CAM or as a quack – if there is no potential patient. And as medical anthropologists keep demonstrating, patients and their families are indeed active in their pursuit of better health. As consumers or "stakeholders" in the pluralistic medical market place they may vote with their feet, seeking out particular healers and demanding specific service provisions. Following from this, a currently prominent theme in western countries is "integrative medicine", which is concerned with how the patients' needs can be satisfied in

12   Kleinman (1998).

a professional and ethically sound manner and health services devised that cater for patients' tendency to "healer hop" or consult treatment providers from a variety of different healing paradigms. There is an ambition to move beyond the internecine warfare between mainstream and CAMs that characterised earlier decades such as the 1960s and 1970s – in some countries notably more so than in others. How does the patient figure in the flow charts of clinical research groups and modern health service providers?

The chart below is from Sweden and focuses on the "Key Processes" or research group activities (P) and the "Structures" or organisational elements (S) created by a research group working on the adaptation of the model of "integrative medicine" to the Swedish primary care context. One question to be asked is how easily we can spot the patient in this diagram.

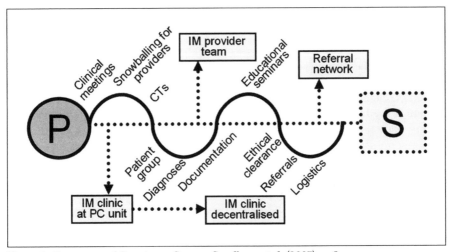

Figure 1: Processes and Structures. Source: Sundberg et al. (2007), p. 3.

The figure refers to the "patient group", lined up alongside other factors such as diagnoses, documentation, ethical clearance, referrals and logistics. The patient is clearly allocated a subordinate role within the processes and structures that characterise this model. Luckily, the Swedish research group developed another chart, which purports to clarify how the patient is supposed to figure in the wider scheme of "integrative medicine" or, as the researchers put it, in a "clinical case management flowchart" (see Figure 2, below).

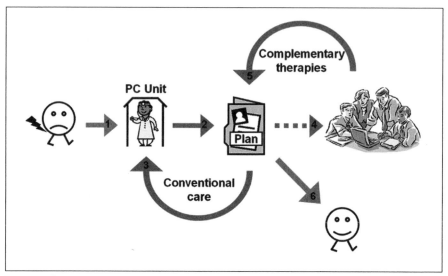

Figure 2: Outcome, the integrative medicine model. Source: Sundberg et al. (2007), p. 6.

Whether the chart indeed clarifies particularly well what is being done to the patient is up for debate. The general idea seems to be: unhappy patient in – happy patient out. What is happening to the patient in between is less clear. Let us see if the further explanations that are provided by the research group help us understand the main processes captured in the model [emphases below are added; WE]:

The integrative medicine model adapted to Swedish primary care illustrated as a clinical case management flowchart:

1) The patient with sub-acute to chronic low back pain or neck pain consults the general practitioner **gatekeeper** at the primary care unit;
2) The patient **and** the general practitioner develop a treatment plan;
3) The patient is **offered** conventional care, i.e. treatment **as usual**;
4) Should complementary therapies **be considered appropriate**, these are integrated into the treatment plan by way of a **consensus case conference** with the integrative medicine provider team;
5) The patient is **offered** complementary therapies as part of the treatment plan, i.e. integrative care;
6) When the treatment plan is completed the case management is finished. **Please note that integrative care was only delivered for up to 12 weeks.**[13]

This Swedish model of integrative medicine in primary care and many others like it are not altogether unproblematic. Where exactly could an active agent be located on the map of pluralistic service provision? We can see the patient at the beginning and at the end, but not anywhere in between. Is the patient being "processed"? How can a self-willed, dynamic factor be fitted in, allo-

---

13   Sundberg et al. (2007), p. 6.

cated a place, and "framed" – perhaps in the double sense of the term – within the wider context of state regulations and the bureaucratic machineries of professionally vetted and ethically and clinically sound user services? Who drives these kinds of through flows of patients? The conventional doctor? The "IMMPT", which is short for "integrative medicine model provider team"? The health service accountant or research administrator who decides on the length of treatment? The patient? In terms of the language employed in the Swedish model, the conventional practitioner clearly remains the "gatekeeper" – in relation to both patient and IMMPT: the patient is being "offered" conventional treatment first and CAM second, and CAM approaches and their practitioners are being integrated into the treatment plan only if judged "appropriate" by the general practitioner.

It seems that despite the recent attempts to shift attention from "medicine" and "practitioner" to "the patient" as the main subject at the heart of medical pluralism, the patient still emerges – usually as an individual rather than within his or her family or other relevant community contexts – as no less elusive in most of the newly designed clinical service settings than patients and families have continued to be in most historical accounts. Paradoxically, the recognition that patients are active agents whose health behaviours tend to cut across disciplinary boundaries and institutional networks has not prevented the reincarnation of Parson's passive "patient role" within the administrative schedules of integrative and supposedly patient-centred medicine.

In regard to the role of CAM practitioners within the integrative medicine model, their integration may well be considered a step forward from earlier opposition and hostility on the part of conventional practitioners some 20 years or so ago. As Kaptchuk and Miller put it: "Opposition, the traditional ethical position that the medical profession must eradicate unconventional medicine for the good of the patient, has withered away."[14] However, they rightly highlight also the major pitfall of integration, which is that it is being achieved on the terms set by conventional medicine. Like many other practitioners, Kaptchuk and Miller therefore champion the principles of patient autonomy and cooperation between and the integrity of conventional as well as CAM approaches. How these principles can be fitted into flow charts and service provision remains an open question.

Plurality and Pluralism

There is the danger of re-objectifying and "passive-ying" patients by the very means intended to chart the channels of patients' shifting preferences and multiple treatment choices from a pluralistic field of health care provisions. The "patient's view" is clearly not the same as viewing the patient. Arguably, CAM practitioners do not fare much better as they still figure as the poorer

---

14   Kaptchuk/Miller (2005), p. 286.

cousin of state-sponsored orthodoxy or adjuncts and accessories to the default setting of conventional care or "treatment as usual". Health policies continue *de facto* to favour the vantage point and methodologies of particular professional interest groups, despite acknowledgement of medical pluralism, which, misteadingly, enunciates for many the idea of equitable coexistence of ideas and practices alongside and complementing each other. The ways in which the maps of medical plurality are drawn in various European countries, the United States, and to a certain extent also in Asia, remain indebted to the predominance of the conventional medicine paradigm, which continues to define the conceptual grid and methodological parameters within which other approaches and the patient are to be located.

Paradoxically, an emphasis on medical plurality and on patients' tendency to healer and paradigm "hop" constitutes both an important corrective to and a reminder of how relevant Foucaultian issues of biopolitics and its *Körpertechniken* continue to be. In the former sense the talk of medical plurality constitutes, as Walach has noted, a thorn in the side of orthodoxy.[15] Rallying around the bandwagon of medical plurality enables CAM practitioners to remind conventional medicine of the popularity of heterodox approaches and the need to reserve a space for the latter lest patients vote with their feet. Therefore, to those faced with the continued biomedical domination via the integration of CAM into the conventional structures of healing on the terms set by medical orthodoxy, mulish insistence by CAMs practitioners on plurality constitutes a means by which to shirk such domination.

At this point the clarification of the terms of reference is called for. How can we conceptually grasp the kind of understanding of medical plurality mooted by CAM practitioners in contrast to the one employed by conventional doctors? Here it may be useful to differentiate the notion of medical plurality from the concept of medical pluralism. The tenets of pluralism enunciate the ideology of a kind of modern liberal heaven where all are equal – but some remain more equal than others. Plurality, in contrast, circumscribes a variety or multitude. It may be argued that issues of definition are trivial farfetched wordplay. However, as Heidegger has stressed, "the word is the house or home of being". Terms such as plurality and pluralism – or nation and nationalism – enunciate related though vitally different phenomena. The "isms" enunciate ideologies. This does not mean that plurality and nation are necessarily devoid of imbalances of power. Rather they may not always be adequately grasped in reference to one particular, period-specific mechanism of legitimating power imbalances, such as pluralism.

"Pluralism" indeed has a chequered history, linked, as it is, to the rise of liberalism in the west – a history of contradictions and controversy in the wake of the European Enlightenment and the unfolding of capitalist society. Although aspired to by liberals intent on doing away with dogma, inequality, patronage and "preferentialism", pluralism has a more sinister side as it is also

---

15   See Walach's essay in this volume.

referred to in contexts characterised by structural inequity. In the latter case, the appeal to pluralism in society has been instrumental in the cover up if not reification of power imbalances, even the sidelining, subordination or subjugation of particular strands of thought, practices and communities' expression of their individual identities. Pluralist societies are not aloof from power politics and hegemonies; they can be a hotbed of them.

To a certain extent, the insistence on differentiating medical plurality and pluralism has its counterpart in more recent concerns about the use of the language of "the medical market" in historical writing. As in the case of medical pluralism, reference to terms such as "supply and demand", "free markets", "commercialisation" and "consumer society" are appropriate only in regard to a particular period, i.e. when the phenomena enshrined in them emerged during the modern period. Gentilcore and Jütte, in their work on healers in pre-modern Italy and Germany respectively, focused on "healing communities" and the openness of and fluidity between specific medical approaches in order to accommodate period-specific concerns and dimensions.[16] They emphasise that the language and notions of the market and pluralism sit uneasily and inappropriately alongside notions of religion, magic, guilds, charity and corporatist structures.

Despite such concerns, the terms medical pluralism and medical market have been used by historians in a merely descriptive way in relation to a variety of historical and geographic contexts to capture the pluralistic and economic aspects of medical practices respectively. Therefore, as pointed out by Jenner and Wallis in relation to market terminology, "its meaning has become vague to the point of confusion".[17] More importantly, its rise during the 1980s characterises late twentieth-century political preoccupations with the ideologies of free markets and the rollback of the state in particular European countries and in North America. The use of market and, arguably, pluralism terminology in historical analyses may therefore be woefully "presentist". Greater precision in the application of enduringly fashionable terms and awareness of their historical and ideological legacies is required lest medical historians mistake historiographic for historical phenomena.

Plural Medicine

In the 1990s, the renowned German philosopher of hermeneutics, Hans-Georg Gadamer, published "The Enigma of Health".[18] He argued that healing is akin not to science but to art, whereby the practitioner is a facilitator who merely helps the patient to "find their own, independent way" on the path to

16 Gentilcore (1998); Jütte (1991).
17 Jenner/Wallis (2007), p. 2. See also Pelling (2009), p. 343.
18 The work was not widely received in English-speaking countries, although a translation was made available in 1996. Gadamer (1996).

recovery from illness.[19] According to Gadamer even modern biomedicine consequently finds itself in "an exceptional and problematic position" *vis-à-vis* other forms of knowledge, with practitioners being pulled in the two different directions of growing scientific rationalization on the one hand and the patient-focused delivery of prudential, personalised treatment on the other.[20] In Gadamer's understanding medicine is practised in a multitude of ways, as successful practitioners will not only interpret and implement medical theories and learned dogma in varied ways but also adapt them to suit different kinds of patients. Within this framework, health and, by implication, medicine are necessarily what I would call "plural".[21] There is a difference between "plural medicine" and both "medical plurality" and "pluralism". Plural medicine signifies that medicine *per se* is always intrinsically "plural", both in terms of the variety of ways in which any one tradition has been interpreted and codified by different learned authorities, and in terms of the great variety of their practical applications.

Seeing any medical approach as plural in itself is particularly relevant in relation to the conference "Medical Pluralism – Past and Present". Here the focus was on medical traditions with a strong literary heritage or grounded in a historical canon of medical texts and therapeutic practices, which despite many changes and transformations retain their value as formative elements of socio-cultural identity. This is particularly relevant in relation to what is often referred to as "indigenous" healing practices common in specific regions, such as Ayurveda, Unani and Siddha in South Asia, for example. Such "traditional" Asian practices have become part of the CAM field of healing in western countries in a multitude of modified and re-imagined versions that better suit the needs of European and American patients. In the history of medicine the focus has usually been on the transfer and dissemination of the western medical model from the west to the east. While this may have been the case in relation to developments during the age of western imperialism, from at least the late twentieth century onwards the globalisation of medical practices has not been a mere one-way traffic. Ayurveda, for example, has been "exported" to the west from India and subsequently re-imported, as its newly westernized and various New Age forms appeal to a largely urban, cosmopolitan elite. Westernized New Age Ayurveda has also been modified further and re-imagined to better resonate with local needs and perceptions in India. These processes of re-invention and re-imaginings have received much attention recently, with earlier concepts such as "hybridization" being replaced with those of the "vernacularization" of, and circulation, crossover and entanglement between, varied medical approaches.

Neither the currently fashionable conceptualization of "indigenous" healing practices as dynamic and subject to globalisation, localisation and re-localisation, nor the phenomenon itself are new in the sense of being a specifically

---

19   Gadamer (1996), p. 109. "Treatment always also involves a certain granting of freedom."
20   Gadamer (1996), pp. 32–33, 39; see also Dallmayr (2000).
21   Ernst (2002).

modern or recent phenomenon. The phenomenon of "vernacularization" of approaches originating in Europe has been traced for both heterodox and orthodox medicine. For example, in my work on mesmerism in British India during the early nineteenth century, I have shown how an approach considered as heterodox (even fraudulent) in Britain was introduced by a Scottish Presbyterian doctor to hospitals and lunatic asylums in Bengal. Here it was adapted with great success to local requirements by his Indian subordinate staff.[22] And Mukharji has shown that even conventional western medicine underwent reconfiguration and was being "vernacularized" or adapted to the socio-cultural needs of patients and practitioners in late nineteenth and early twentieth-century India in the shape of "Daktari" medicine.[23] Clearly, earlier historians' focus on East-West and North-South divides and on one-way transfer and the globalisation of the western medicine paradigm has been superseded by increased emphasis on local modifications and adaptations and on the links and exchanges between nations and localities across the globe.[24]

One persistently contentious issue concerns the point that there may be disagreements among and between scholars and practitioners about which one of the many kinds of Ayurveda, for example, might be closest to any supposedly "original" blueprint. Would it be appropriate to assume that those practices mentioned in the ancient Indian Vedic texts, for example, are the truly authentic ones, preferable to the practices and procedures focused on in modern-day Ayurveda? And, if so, which one of these, out of an array of different textual traditions, would we choose as the definite source? Even if there was such a thing as an original blueprint of *the* Ayurvedic doctrine, would it make sense to elevate the written tradition above Ayurvedic doctors' real-life, and usually more "messy" and idiosyncratic, practical adaptations and modifications of the theoretical corpus? And what about patients' active role in the pursuit of better health and consumers' decision in favour of medical approaches that appeal to them on account of their perceived authenticity and anticipated benefit? Does it matter that current representations and practices of particular approaches are relatively recent re-inventions of tradition (as in the case of Traditional Chinese Medicine[25]) or akin to modern re-imaginings on the basis of current needs (as in modern Yoga, for example[26]), and therefore at times but faintly linked with any one of the various brands of medicine practised in South Asia or China centuries ago? Ultimately, the question arises of how we could define, delimit and "frame" any one particular medical approach if we think of them as intrinsically plural and therefore as perceived and practised in a dynamic, versatile and pluralistic way in different locations and points in time – in South Asia and China as much as in Europe and North America.

22 Ernst (2004).
23 Mukharji (2009).
24 See, for example: Ernst/Mueller (2010); Digby/Ernst/Mukharji (2010).
25 Scheid (2002).
26 Ernst (2003).

Conclusion

Historians of medicine have begun to recognize the importance of transnational links, circulation of ideas and practices, and the globalisation of western as well as indigenous medicines. Such work focuses on the plurality of approaches and the intrinsically plural nature of healing, emphasizing processes of vernacularization on account of practitioners' virtuosity in adapting their approach to particular patient groups and moving between different doctrines, as well as patients' versatility as they healer and "cosmology hop" and draw on a number of different strands of medical practices. Nevertheless, the "patient's view" remains conspicuous by its continued absence in most medical histories, with patient-focused accounts mapping patients' choices rather than their perceptions and experiences of particular medical paradigms. Despite the recent trend towards patient-centred and integrative medicine, both patients and CAM practitioners remain subjugated to the concerns of and control by conventional medicine and health service providers. This is only to be expected within socio-economic and political structures currently dominated by the free market premises and the concept of pluralism. However, while medical pluralism in the modern period may be adequately configured as subject to market forces, the applicability of market and pluralism terminology to pre-modern and non-western manifestations of medical plurality needs to be questioned. Such an understanding would not only avoid anachronistic accounts of pre-modern and non-western healing but also open awareness of the historical contingency and therefore the scope for change of modern conceptual frameworks.

Bibliography

Attewell, Guy: Refiguring Unani *tibb*. Plural Healing in Late-colonial India. New Delhi 2007.
Cant, Sarah; Sharma, Ursula: A new medical Pluralism? Alternative medicine, doctors, patients and the state. London 1999.
Dallmayr, Fred: "The Enigma of Health": Hans-Georg Gadamer at 100. In: The Review of Politics 62 (2000), no. 2, pp. 327–350.
Digby, Anne; Ernst, Waltraud; Mukharji, Projit B. (eds.): Crossing Colonial Historiographies. Histories of Colonial and Indigenous Medicines in Transnational Perspective. Newcastle 2010.
Dinges, Martin (ed.): Patients in the History of Homoeopathy. Sheffield 2002.
Eguchi, Shigeyuki: Between folk-concepts of illness and psychiatric diagnosis: Kitsune-tsuki (fox possession) in a mountain village of Western Japan. In: Culture, Medicine and Psychiatry 15 (1991), no. 4, pp. 421–451.
Ernst, Waltraud: Plural Medicine, Tradition and Modernity. Historical and Contemporary perspectives: views from below and from above. In: Ernst, Waltraud (ed.): Plural Medicine, Tradition and Modernity, 1800–2000. London; New York 2002, pp. 1–18.
Ernst, Waltraud: Cultural Import – Yoga, Plural Medicine and East-West Exchanges. In: Arnold, Ken; Boon, Tim (eds.): Treat Yourself. London 2003, pp. 12–14.
Ernst, Waltraud: Colonial psychiatry, magic and religion. The case of mesmerism in British India. In: *History of Psychiatry* 15 (2004), no. 1, pp. 57–71.

Ernst, Waltraud: Beyond East and West. From the History of Colonial Medicine to a Social History of Medicine(s) in South Asia. In: Social History of Medicine 20 (2007), pp. 505–524.

Ernst, Waltraud; Mueller, Thomas (eds.): Transnational Psychiatries. Social and Cultural Histories of Psychiatry in Comparative Perspective, c. 1800–2000. Newcastle 2010.

Etsuko, Matsuoka: The interpretation of fox possession: Illness as metaphor. In: Culture, Medicine and Psychiatry 15 (1991), no. 4, pp. 453–477.

Gadamer, Hans-Georg: The Enigma of Health: The Art of Healing in a Scientific Age. Stanford 1996.

Gentilcore, David: Healers and Healing in Early Modern Italy. Manchester 1998.

Jenner, Mark; Wallis, Patrick (eds.): Medicine and the Market in England and its Colonies, c. 1450–1850. Basingstoke 2007.

Jütte, Robert: Ärzte, Heiler und Patienten: medizinischer Alltag in der frühen Neuzeit. München; Zürich 1991.

Kaptchuk, Ted J.; Eisenberg, David M.: Varieties of Healing. 1: Medical Pluralism in the United States. In: Annals of Internal Medicine 135 (2001), no. 3, pp. 189–195.

Kaptchuk, Ted J.; Miller, Franklin G.: What is the Best and Most Ethical Model for the Relationship Between Mainstream and Alternative Medicine: Opposition, Integration, or Pluralism? In: Academic Medicine 80 (2005), no. 3, pp. 286–290.

Kleinman, Arthur: The illness narratives: suffering, healing, and the human condition. New York 1998.

Matthiessen, Peter F.: Paradigmenpluralität und Individualmedizin. In: Matthiessen, Peter F. (ed.): Patientenorientierung und Professionalität. Bad Homburg 2010, pp. 87–113.

Mukharji, Projit B.: Nationalizing the Body. The Medical Market, Print and Daktari Medicine. New York 2009.

Pelling, Margaret: Medical Conflicts in Early Modern London: Patronage, Physicians, and Irregular Practitioners 1550–1640. Oxford 2009.

Porter, Roy: The Patient's View: Doing Medical History from Below. In: Theory and Society 14 (1985), pp. 175–198.

Scheid, Volker: Chinese Medicine in Contemporary China. Plurality and Synthesis. Durham; London 2002.

Scheper-Hughes, Nancy: The madness of hunger: Sickness, delirium, and human needs. In: Culture, Medicine and Psychiatry 12 (1988), no. 4, pp. 429–458.

Sundberg, Tobias et al.: Towards a model for integrative medicine in Swedish primary care. In: Biomed Central Health Services Research 7 (2007), no. 107, available on: http://www.biomedcentral.com/content/pdf/1472-6963-7-107.pdf (accessed 5 Dec. 2012).

Medical Pluralism in Early Modern Germany

Robert Jütte

The proto-professionalization of health care

In the long drawn-out conflict between the representatives of "academic" medicine on the one hand and "empirical" medicine on the other a hierarchical health system evolved in early modern Germany and other European countries. The conflict was not just about competition for patients but also about the capacity for medical interpretation. At the top of the hierarchy were the university-trained physicians, followed in turn by apothecaries, barbers, surgeons and midwives. What they all had in common was that they were officially licensed to practise their professions.[1]

Far into early modern times the plague and other epidemics constituted the greatest challenge for individuals as well as authorities.[2] First in Italy and then also in German cities a sanitary instrumentarium (from hygiene to quarantine) was tested with more or less success and approved.[3] As a result the health-care system was thoroughly transformed. Health and illness were no longer a private but a public matter.[4] Once this view had taken root, it was only a small step to the "medical police" of the seventeenth and eigthteenth centuries that was later to be replaced by another paradigm, that of "social medicine".[5] If it had not been for the continuous fear of epidemics the members of the medical fraternity would have struggled to gain priority over their "competitors" in the healing trade. Which is not to say that physicians, a few exceptions granted, were particularly prominent in the care and treatment of plague victims. On the contrary, their popularity was rather limited since many of them had preferred to flee to the relative safety of the country rather than remain in the plague-ridden towns. Nevertheless, at least the authorities listened to their political health care advisers and heeded the counsel of the physicians in whom they had put their trust. How much they were appreciated is obvious from the fact that in the seventeenth and eighteenth centuries

---

1   For studies on health care in early modern German cities, see: Steinhilber (1956); Gensthaler (1973); Weingärtner (1981); Knefelkamp (1981); Schwanitz (1990); Jütte (1991); Eckardt (1991); Wolfgang Fischer (1991); Münkle (1992); Krauß (1993); Neubrand (1994); Müller (1994); Kinzelbach (1995); Plank (1999); Hammond (2000). For regional studies, see: Jäck/Nauck (1951); Terhalle (1965); Watermann (1977); Wischhöfer (1991); Loetz (1993); Lindemann (1996).
2   Cf. Cipolla (1973); Dinges (1995).
3   Cf. Dinges (1994); Dinges (1995).
4   Cf. Jütte: Gesundheitsverständnis (2008).
5   Cf. Rosen (1974). See also Schwartz (1973); Frevert (1984); Dinges (2000); Wahrig/Sohn (2003); Möller (2005).

a growing number of academically trained physicians were assigned seats and votes on political committees.[6]

The plague epidemics – though catastrophic from a demographic point of view – exemplify how the health-care system reacts to influences from the outside and adapts to a new situation by bestowing on one particular group the monopoly to interpret what illness is and how it is to be remedied. In the last three decades, studies on the social history of medicine have shown how social, economic, political and technological developments also induced and effected changes in the medical system of a society.[7]

Demand and supply in the early modern health market

Let us now look at the inner structure of the health-care system and at its users. In all societies the primary experience of needing and receiving help has brought about basic patterns of coping with illness individually and collective-ly.[8] This anthropological model of medical care-giving applies equally to modern, traditional or pre-industrial societies and can be used in socio-histor-ical analysis of early modern health care. Medical systems are, in principle, the same everywhere, they do, however, generate different surface structures depending on the given social and cultural environment. Arthur Kleinman, in his fundamental ethno-medical studies[9], separates the system of medical health care into three sectors that cannot exist independently of each other. They overlap when patients – as often happens – receive medical help succes-sively or simultaneously from family members, a physician or a faith healer while assuming the role of sick relative, patient or client respectively.

Folk medicine, often referred to as "lay medicine", has always been a highly important and often underrated form of collective self-help. Its services and functions include the use of lay knowledge that has been tested and "proved", the sharing of experience, information and remedies, the referral of patients to competent helpers, the supervision of healers, the provision of care for the sick and for women in childbed. Patients experience their illness within the social group that is closest to them, usually their family. They reveal their symptoms, if they are not self-evident, to their relatives. The family assigns to them the role of patients, arranges for the necessary medical help and nursing and participates in the decision as to the success of the treatment and the choice of therapeutic alternatives. Folk medicine can therefore be described as the "management of episodes of illness and critical life situations with the re-

6   On membership of physicians in German town councils, see Herborn (1985), pp. 357ff.; Kintzinger (2000), pp. 76–77.
7   See, for example, Risse (1979).
8   See, for instance, Seidler (1978).
9   Kleinman (1980), p. 50, figure 3.

sources provided by the social environment".[10] It is obvious that the social system in question is strengthened in the process.

It would be wrong to place today's "professionalized" health service on a par with the pre-industrial medical system that, though well organised, was rather "semi-professional" in many respects. The old, historically grown complexity endured far into the nineteenth century and it took several reform attempts to define the boundaries between the various medical areas of competence and to ensure their observance. Only gradually did the "collegia medica" emerge, representing the academically qualified physicians who aspired to a monopoly in medicine.[11] The barbers and surgeons were able to maintain their traditionally strong position in the healing hierarchy until the nineteenth century when they were gradually pushed out of the health market as providers of surgical interventions.[12] They were replaced by academically trained surgeons who were the first to benefit from the "professionalization" that was promoted by the authorities.[13] It was similar for midwives who were gradually superseded by male "specialists"[14], but different for pharmacists who succeeded in maintaining their status for centuries although they were not safe from the "professionalization" process either[15]. Since the late Middle Ages their function had been clearly defined and restricted to the manufacture and sale of medicines according to a physician's prescription, but it took a long time for the state to actually enforce the observation of such restrictions.

The road to "a distinction of rank, the setting up of a self-regulation mechanism, the cultivation of prestige"[16] was long and winding. This goal was prepared in medieval and early modern times[17] through the teaching of a Greek-Arabic curriculum at universities, which was eventually, through various intermediary stages and transformations, transmitted from the academic physicians to the medical lay system[18]. The physicians, and to some extent also the surgeons, increasingly assumed public functions as supervisors and inspectors of the other healing professions and took on the tasks of a health police (policing of epidemics, forensic medicine). Their commitment to a "professionalism" that befitted their rank became manifest early on in the professional oath of master and student surgeons and the hippocratic oath. A canon of indepen-

10 Dornheim (1986), p. 17.
11 Cf. Alfons Fischer (1933), vol. 1, p. 329. For case studies, see Klimpel (1995); Gossmann (1966); Münch (1995).
12 Cf. Sander (1989).
13 See Groß (1999).
14 Cf., for example, Gabler (1985); Loytved (2001); Blankenburg (2003); Stadlober-Degwerth (2008); Schaffer/Werner (2009); Seidel (1998).
15 Friedrich/Müller-Jahncke (2005), pp. 189ff.
16 Schipperges (1978), p. 463.
17 Cf. Bullough (1966).
18 Cf. Schenda (1982); MacLean (2002); Horn/Dorffner/Eichinger (2007); Dinges/Jütte (2011).

dent, specialist literature (textbooks, polemic writings against charlatanism, expert opinions) was generated.[19]

In medieval and early modern times the boundary between "folk medicine" and university-taught medicine was still diffuse and vague despite the vehement delimitation efforts of the medical fraternity. This only changed in the Age of Enlightenment when academic and popular medicine began to separate. Due to the progress achieved by the increasingly empirical natural sciences (physics and chemistry in particular) new successful therapies were discovered: "Popular beliefs were no longer of relevance to physicians."[20] The gulf between the two medical cultures widened and became ultimately unbridgeable.[21]

In early modern times empirical and religious-magic elements often came together in therapy.[22] It still makes sense to differentiate between "magic medicine" and "empirical medicine".[23] Empirical medicine is based on experience and comprises a great number of "natural medicines" that had "proved" their worth over the centuries. Scholarly physicians referred as "empirics" to all those who had not undergone academic training, including Jewish physicians. They considered them to be incapable of understanding the effect of the remedies they prescribed because they lacked "eruditio" and "doctrina".[24] The difference between empirical medicine and the Hippocratic-Galenic medicine that was taught at universities was mostly superficial: academic physicians tended to prescribe the same remedies but thought it essential to know something about causality. Ideas we would today refer to the realm of sympathetic magic or folk beliefs (for instance that lungwort can cure lung disease because of its shape) used to belong to "rational" medicine up to the eighteenth century. "Rational" meant not only knowing the cause of a disease but also "the remedies of which experience taught us that they were sent for this purpose [...]".[25] Human skin, for instance, was an unusual but certainly "natural" remedy that had nothing to do with white magic as it was understood at the time, because one knew from experience how it worked and was in possession of a suitable causal medical theory. When in 1609 the Munich executioner Hans Stadler was accused of using magic, he pointed out in his defence that he only employed natural remedies such as herbs, roots and human tallow.[26] The fact that early modern official pharmacopoeias listed parts of the dead human body proves that they were thought to have a "natural" remedial effect. Treatments by executioners with human tallow and skin from corpses were therefore rational in the sense of the then prevailing humoral medicine, but also in

19 See, for example, Walter (2008).
20 Diepgen (1967), p. 213.
21 Cf. Stenzel (2005).
22 Cf. Müller-Jahncke (1985).
23 See, for example, Jütte: Geschichte (1996), pp. 66ff.
24 Cf. Elkeles (1987). On stereotypes regarding Jewish doctors, see Hortzitz (1994); Jütte: Zur Funktion (1996).
25 J. G. Krüger, Naturlehre (1765), quoted in Witzel (1990), p. 35.
26 See, for example, Jütte: Menschliche Gewebe (2008).

the sense of Paracelsus' natural philosophical ideas that continued to be very popular in the eighteenth century.

It is different with the kind of magic that shares little common ground with scientific medicine. It is not based on experience or reality but believes in a mysterious relationship between the disease and the sensory or supersensory world and tries to cure disease with magic. Although it makes sense to differentiate beween empirical and magic medicine for terminological reasons, the boundaries between the two were fluid in early modern times, as Irmgard Hampp pointed out: "You find prescriptions for the use of herbs and the manufacture of ointments and potions on the same page as magic spells against diseases and instructions for mysterious acts of magic. This shows that what we know as folk medicine was based as much on empiricism as on magic."[27]

Especially the church had its difficulties with the magic elements of folk medicine over the centuries, because "what the church sees as 'superstition', is [...] not just pure magic but mostly magic intermingled with religious elements."[28] The Catholic and Protestant churches considered magic healing to be incompatible with the Christian faith.[29] Catholic theologians, moreover, were continually faced with the problem of having to separate the widespread pagan belief in demons and sympathetic magic used in healing from "spiritual remedies" such as exorcism, pilgrimages, votive offerings and intercessions. What the dogmatists thought out had usually little to do with reality. Even after the reformation and the Tridentine Reforms we find evidence that many priests were not quite sure of the line between magic and the legitimate Christian belief in miracles.[30]

With so much variety on offer in the health market, competition was rife among the healers in early modern cities. The surgeons in Cologne, for instance, not only complained about unfair competition among their colleagues, but increasingly expressed their displeasure at the foreign "charlatans". The apothecaries also vied for potential clients, as the number of pharmacies was indeed astounding. In the sixteenth century, Cologne boasted one pharmacy per 2634 citizens (slightly less than in Germany today!). It is therefore not surprising that in the seventeenth century Cologne City Council did all it could to limit the number of pharmacies to twelve to make sure that all apothecaries had a sufficient and appropriate income.[31] We unfortunately have no comparative sources for that time with regard to registered midwives[32] but we

---

27 Hampp (1961), p. 32.
28 Hampp (1961), p. 12.
29 Cf. Thomas (1988); Grell/Cunningham (2007).
30 Cf. Signori (2007), especially O'Neill (1984).
31 See, for example, Historical Archives of the City of Cologne (HAStK), Verfassung und Verwaltung (VuV), Nachträge 89 (7.7.1674); Ratsprotokolle 111, f. 237v (4.11.1665); Ratsprotokolle 113, f. 245r (18.10.1666). See also Schmidt (1931), p. 70, who explains the high number of apothecaries in Cologne with additional business activities (e.g. spice trade).
32 See, for example, Boventer (1976), p. 78. According to Wiesner (1986), p. 59, the number of midwives varied from town to town in the 16th century: Strasbourg (6), Augsburg (19),

can assume that Cologne, just as other German cities, had one midwife for approximately every 1500 inhabitants.

To this large number of approved urban healers we have to add the diverse lay-healers, who were then, as they are now, very popular with patients. It is difficult to make a quantitative statement with regard to this rather significant segment of urban health care, as unlicensed healers were not usually registered.

Before we briefly introduce, based on the imperial city of Cologne, the individual sectors of the official and other health-care systems, let us look at where the "providers" were located. Socio-topographical investigation into early modern health care is unfortunately still scarce in the German-speaking realm, which means that we do not know how typical the situation in Cologne was of other towns of that time.[33]

The parishes of Klein St Martin, St Brigiden, St Alban and St Kolumba boasted a particularly high proportion of healers (measured by the number of households). The Cologne "health market" was therefore mostly concentrated around the Roman centre, in what is today the historic town. As with many other trades, it was not irrelevant for the various healing professionals where they practised. With the exception of the apothecaries – since the Middle Ages most pharmacies in Cologne were situated around the historic market (*Alter Markt*)[34] – the health professionals had no preferred location, but practising physicians, barbers and midwives nevertheless made sure that there were enough clients close to their place of residence or practice. This view is not only supported by the topographical map [Fig. 1] and also by occasional archival indications that explicitly describe how a surgeon, for instance, relocated to another parish because of the lack of patients in his former place of residence.[35] Most Cologne parishes had at least one barber, surgeon or midwife[36] while the few academically trained physicians and the numerous apothecaries preferred to be close to the university (the arts and law faculties), grammar schools and the wealthy monasteries, especially the *Domstift* (Cathedral chapter). The area along the Rhine was obviously also sought after, because it was the first port of call for strangers who arrived by boat. It is not surprising that apothecaries, barbers and formally trained physicians preferred to settle along the main traffic arteries. In the parish of St Kolumba, in the *Breite Straße* and *Schildergasse* (both vital thoroughfares and trunk roads to the East and West), we mostly find representatives of the "official" medicine (among them a "medicus", four surgeons and a midwife).

Memmingen (2–5), Frankfurt am Main (6–12).

33   Jütte (1989), p. 30.
34   See Schmidt (1931), p. 26f.
35   See, for example, HAStK, VuV, G 261 (8.2.1652).
36   For a similar pattern, see Pelling (1986), p. 87.

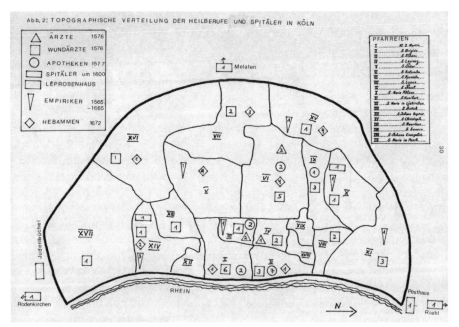

Figure 1: Topographical map of Cologne

The relationship between "rich" and "poor" parishes and the urban healing hierarchy is not quite as unambiguous. Due to a lack of sources relating to early modern times we have no information on the distribution of wealth among Cologne's citizens. An incomplete "chimney tax register" from 1582 provides one clue.[37] A high proportion of the healing community practised in parishes where almost one third of the recorded citizens paid tax for more than four chimneys and where the number of poor households was below three per cent. There was one exception to this rule: in the parish of St Aposteln almost three quarters of tax payers lived in houses or flats with only one chimney, but the parish had at times three resident barbers and the same number of midwives. That the spread of healers in early modern towns was not accidental is evident from the location of two Cologne hospitals: *Revilien* and *Weite Tür*. One was in the Northern part of the town, the other in the South so that maids and servants, who had to carry patients to hospital when required, did not have to cover such long distances. The four leper infirmaries were banished to locations outside the town walls for health-political reasons. The same applied to the plague house which was set up – against the expressed wishes and under the protest of residents – in front of *Kunibertsturm* (Kunibert Tower), that is outside the parish gates where the houses stood less closely together.[38]

37   See Jütte (1984), pp. 227ff.
38   Cf. Mering (1857), p. 152.

Competitors in the early modern health market

In rank and reputation, the formally educated physicians occupied the very top of the medical hierarchy and differed clearly from other licensed practitioners (surgeons, barber-surgeons, apothecaries, midwives) who had not been to medical school. There were, however, relatively few such physicians at that time. In 1576 Cologne had only eight physicians. Some of them died within a year without having successors lined up to take over their practice or their teaching commitments at the medical school. Shortly before he himself passed away on 8 June 1576, Dr Hermann Kollenberg, private physician to the Weinsberg family, offered his lapidary comment on the high number of deaths among his colleagues: "Doctors do not grow very old" ("Die medici worden nit seir alt").[39] The medical fraternity was indeed short of successors because physicians, who wanted to practise in the city, not only had to present a master's degree from the philosophical faculty, they also had to have earned their doctorate in Cologne *"more majorum"*, i.e. in an immensely expensive and highly ceremonial procedure. For a lecturing post at the university a one-off payment of 100 Florin was sufficient and no expensive "doctors' dinner" was needed. It also earned the candidate a doctoral title but only *"per modum transeuntis"*. As a rule, medical students had to study for three years to gain the bachelor degree and a further two years for the licentiate, for which a compulsory curriculum existed (mainly consisting of the writings of Hippocrates and Galen). In a final examination candidates had to defend their medical thesis. They had to swear under oath that they were not excommunicated, married or dishonourable and that they were not practising surgeons or murderers.[40] Over and above that, newly qualified licentiates had to promise never to practise together with Jews, untrained men or women. If their tasks should require it, they were permitted to consult and accept the help of experienced and confirmed surgeons. If they wanted to obtain a doctorate as well, they had to pay dearly for the privilege, as described earlier, and they had to attend further lectures. If the medical faculty permitted it at all, they could practise within a six-mile radius of the city during that period and for the first year they could only attend the sick if they were accompanied by their supervisor. An entry in the council minutes from 1656 shows, however, that the members of the medical faculty were not overly concerned with the visiting of patients: professors had to be admonished not to "leave any patients without comfort by neglecting to visit and treat them".[41] Especially during the plague the medical professors proved rather unreliable, in Cologne as elsewhere. During the epidemic of 1666 many of them fled to the country. Some members of the medical faculty even refused to attend to "contagious" patients once the epi-

---

39 HAStK, Chroniken und Darstellungen 49, f. 719r.
40 See, for example, HAStK, Univ.-Akten 367, f. 38.
41 HAStK, Ratsprotokolle 103, f. 330v.

demic was over, forcing the council to threaten them with suspension from their lecturing post and corresponding loss of income.[42]

Most academic physicians recognized "empirical knowledge" as legitimate as long as it did not call the traditional healing hierarchy into question. This applied to the medical knowledge of surgeons that was passed on within a guild. Surgeons in Cologne and other towns were not allowed to treat internal diseases or prescribe or manufacture laxatives and emetics. The Medical Act of 1628 prescribed in detail what kind of knowledge a practising surgeon needed to acquire. He had to have worked as an apprentice in Cologne for four years and as a journeyman for two more years before he was permitted to practise independently. The knowledge acquired during his years of training included a thorough understanding of the human anatomy, in particular "of the natural difference between the limbs, their constitution and position, and what was to be applied and used at various times to treat wounds, bullet or stab wounds, burns and their concomitants, dislocations, fractures and other damage".[43] Surgeons, such as Wilhelm Fabry in the seventeenth century, who ranked almost as high as academic physicians, were absolute exceptions. The field was dominated by more-or-less experienced surgeons and barber-surgeons of whose social background, education and everyday practice we still have very little knowledge. The academically trained physicians might at times ridicule their lack of theoretical knowledge and reprimand the one or other of them for overstepping his remit, but the patients had so much confidence in them that they simply have to be seen as the true pillars of the early modern medical system.[44]

Within the healing trade, the surgeons were certainly the most prominent group in quantitative terms. During the second half of the fifteenth century, when Cologne had almost 40,000 inhabitants, its barber office (*Barbieramt*), an independent corporation that had existed since 1397, numbered at least 36 members.[45] In the early seventeenth century the cathedral town still had 32 surgeons and barber-surgeons.[46] Some of them only practised in what was termed "half office", which meant they were not allowed to dress wounds on their own or train apprentices. Although the population grew only slowly the number of barber practices rose in the late seventeenth century which made for more intense competition so that Cologne City Council decided in 1714 "that the number of barbers is to be reduced to forty, and that henceforth no well-meant counsel, under whatever pretext, is to be accepted without special permission".[47] Occasional references to other sidelines prove that, even before

---

42 Cf. Keussen (1934), p. 279. For a particular incident, see HAStK, Ratsprotokolle 112, f. 288r.
43 Printed in Schmidt (1931), pp. 113–117. Quotation from article 23.
44 Cf. Neumann (2007), p. 89.
45 For an early list of members, see HAStK, Zunft-Akten 355, f. 73r-74r. Cf. Jütte (1995).
46 See HAStK, Zunft-Akten 355, f. 193r.
47 HAStK, Zunft-Akten 371, p. 407 (28.9.1714).

that, not all barbers had been able to survive only on their income from wound treatment, blood-letting, haircuts and shaving.[48]

Specialists among the surgeons, such as stone and hernia cutters or oculists, were not usually organized in guilds. Among Cologne's resident surgeons there were few specialists for eye problems or inguinal and scrotal hernias. These were difficult procedures that relied on a sure hand and plenty of experience and they were therefore left to the non-resident surgeons who visited the town (not only Cologne) on an irregular basis.[49]

Pharmacies had an important role to play within the official health-care system of Cologne and other early modern towns. Since the "profession of the apothecary is a particularly worthy one, concerning the human body and life, which parish and town have a strong need for and interest in"[50], as it says in a report of the Cologne Medical Faculty from 1478, it was, already in the late Middle Ages, regulated to the last detail by the relevant authorities. Apothecaries increasingly came to be "servants" of university-trained physicians, entrusted merely with the dispensation of remedies. In the fierce competition that arose due to the relatively large number of pharmacies in the sixteenth and seventeenth centuries, not all pharmacists adhered to the rules or official recommendations, since patients were free to "have prescriptions and remedies prepared and manufactured in the pharmacy which they prefer or habitually frequent".[51] It is therefore not surprising that some apothecaries occasionally fulfilled the special wishes of their customers even if it involved bending the rules here or there. Others tried to boost their business by mixing inferior substances into their remedies, hoping that the laymen would not detect the fraud. This is the reason why Cologne physician Bernhard Dessen von Cronenburg suggested to the city's authorities in his book on the composition of remedies (1555) that they should either supervise the apothecaries better or permit the physicians to dispense their own medicines.[52] The City Council of Cologne opted for the first of these suggestions and established an official pharmacy oversight scheme in the second half of the sixteenth century.[53]

According to the Medical Act of the City of Cologne from 1628 – the same applied to other towns, too[54] – midwives had to give evidence of a good reputation and of their "Catholic religion" on top of having to pass an examination in the presence of the Dean of the Medical Faculty[55]. There are in fact occasional references in early modern sources to the effect that midwives did not

---

48 For Freiburg im Breisgau, cf. Knefelkamp (1981), p. 125, footnote 109.
49 Cf., for instance, Hieke (2002); Pies (2004); Hauri (2010).
50 Quoted in Schmidt (1931), p. 105.
51 See Article 5 of the Medical Act of 1628, quoted in Schmidt (1931), pp. 113–114.
52 See Schmidt (1931), p. 42.
53 See, for example, HAStK, Ratsprotokolle 19, f. 304v (3.10.1558), f. 367v (17.4.1559); Ratsprotokolle 56, f. 91v (16.5.1607); Ratsprotokolle 76, f. 212v (1.6.1630). See also HAStK, Edikte 3.48 (23.5.1588).
54 Cf. Schilling (1980); Wiesner (1986), pp. 55ff.
55 Quoted in Schmidt (1931), p. 117.

know enough about anatomy and obstetrics.[56] If one takes into account that midwifery typically relied on "empirical knowledge"[57] it does not come as a surprise that the majority of midwives accused of witchcraft in the early seventeenth century in Cologne, were married, had given birth to several children and were over fifty years old. There was no special training yet for midwives in early modern times. The necessary know-how was passed on by mouth[58] or could be found in vernacular textbooks such as Eustachius Rösslin's "Hebammen Roßgarten" (1513) or his "Ehestandsartzneibuch" (1534).

The emergence of a hierarchy of healers that was promoted by the authorities was accompanied by the growing discrimination against "charlatans" and "quacks". Even before medical law began to accumulate punishments for unlicensed practitioners, the medical literature that was composed by formally trained physicians used strong words to describe the charlatans and their clients, as in the preface to Johannes Dryander's "Practicierbüchlin" (1589):

> We therefore need to proceed with utmost modesty and reason, not to wrongly entrust body and life to untrained hags/ and inexperienced calf doctors, unlearned monks, Jews/ and foolish women, etc. who most likely learned their art haphazardly behind the stove and have the audacity to try it out on me or you like a cobbler who makes shoes for everybody over the same last/ Such vagabonds and cozeners have one remedy, potion, ointment, plaster for all ailments so that many have risked their lives.[59]

The discrimination against medical outsiders by the members of the medical fraternity was pitted against the people's need for help, especially in "hopeless" cases. The Paracelsian Georg Fedro von Rhodach was quick to respond to vicious attacks from Cologne physicians by pointing out that the learned physicians were more often than not at their wit's end: "To this hour I never took on a patient anywhere who had not been discharged as incurable by Galenic doctors/ surgeons and other artists."[60] It is therefore not surprising that "empirics" were not only vastly popular, but often found influential advocates who defended them to the municipal authorities. Even a German emperor occasionally rather heeded the advice of a wise woman than that of a well-remunerated personal physician.[61] Why should his subjects, who could not even afford the high rates of a medicus, act differently?

Unlicensed healers can be divided in two groups. One group whose members "present themselves on the market, or [...] in other places with their quack medicines"[62] is frequently mentioned in medical history. The second group was less conspicuous and therefore of less interest to the history of medicine. Johannes Bohn wrote about members of this group in 1704 that they "boldly practised medicine in an overt or covert way with little or no medical

---

56 See Remmen (1965), pp. 62ff.
57 Cf. Böhme (1981), pp. 457ff.
58 See, for example, HAStK, VuV, G 252, f. 208v (15.3.1631).
59 Dryander (1589), pp. 4–5.
60 Fedro (1566), Sig. Ci (v).
61 For the treatment of Emperor Maximilian II by a "wise woman", see Treue (1955), pp. 329–330.
62 HAStK, Univ.-Akten 450, f. 3.

knowledge, from a permanent place of residence in town or in the country".[63]
At the time it was thought that among these resident practitioners were "not
only common people, old women, priests and doctors, but also apothecaries,
Paracelsians, doctores, who do not know their trade but practise and treat patients on the basis of mere experience or using certain books that offer good
recipes for any illness".[64] Such complaints about travelling quacks but also
about resident "charlatans" are numerous in the literature. These sources are
however not altogether suitable for the reconstruction of this important aspect
of everyday medical culture, because they say more about the relationship
between the members of the medical fraternity and the more-or-less authorized practitioners than about the actual position held by "empirics" within the
health-care system. There are archival sources that are more instructive in this
respect.

In early modern sources we frequently come across resident "quack doctors" who, for one reason or another, were put on record. It can be assumed
that the cases that have become known constitute merely the tip of the iceberg
because members of this group were not usually that conspicuous if they did
not openly perform superstitious practices. Most "empirics" had other jobs as
well which they only very rarely gave up in order to devote themselves to the
more lucrative practice of healing. Some of them possessed a degree of surgical knowledge that they had either gained in an uncompleted apprenticeship
with a barber-surgeon or in the war. In the eyes of the professionals, who were
organized in guilds, they were not much better than lay practitioners who pre-
sumed to cure wounds and ailments.

A special case among the lay healers was a group who also had some practical knowledge of healing. They were the executioners and hangmen. The
society that banished executioners from its midst, branding them as outsiders,
did not scorn their helping hands if they promised healing. As in other cities[65],
the executioner in Cologne had the reputation that he was not only a good
"bonesetter" but also a knowledgeable healer. It is small wonder that these
healers, who were generally very popular despite their dubious origin, were
thorns in the flesh of the physicians and surgeons. Many executioners treated
their patients if not much better so hardly worse than the average surgeon.[66] It
says much about the state of medical science at the time that a man like Paracelsus thought it appropriate to learn not only from travellers and barbers, but
also from executioners.[67]

The "wise women"[68] also belonged to the group of resident empirics, not
least due to their affinity to magic practices. But they were not "honest and

63 Bohn, Johannes: De officio medici duplici [...]. Leipzig 1704, quoted in Elkeles (1987), p.
    200.
64 Horst (1574), p. 10.
65 See, for example, Nowosadtko (1994); Stuart (1999).
66 For a contemporary diatribe, see Hörnigk (1638), p. 187.
67 Cf. Heinemann (1900), p. 8.
68 See, for instance, Wiesner (1986), pp. 49ff.; Ahrendt-Schulte (1994); Rummel (2000).

good women [...] who tended to those in need by providing them with liquor, also boiled potions, juices, electuaries, fruit preserves, and such like out of the goodness of their hearts and without asking for payment"[69], as one contemporary critic of lay-medicine put it. As soon as women overstepped their allocated (domestic) bounds of medical help and care and asked for payment or administered remedies without the supervision and direction of a physician, they were denounced by the "licensed" healers.

The "quack doctors" who travelled from fair to fair, trying to to sell their miracle potions by advertising them vociferously and dramatically, differed from the various resident healers of heterogeneous social standing and education. What both had in common was that they practised to a great extent illegally. However much the general population liked the travelling doctors and remedy sellers because of their allegedly miraculous potions[70], the authorities did not always trust them. They had to meet certain requirements, pay high fees for their stalls and pass the occasional examination in order to obtain the longed-for licence that was usually limited to a short period of time. A council order issued in Cologne in 1614 illustrates the hostility of the municipal decision-makers: it authorized organizers of markets to "remove vagrants, quacks and other idle folk from the market".[71] The combination of medicine and dramatic performance for advertising and business purposes was certainly a thorn in the magistrate's flesh. The relationship between the travelling quack doctors and dabblers and the resident healers was informed by a sense of competition and snobbishness, as one can easily imagine. In 1649 the Cologne surgeons complained about Johann Potage that he "sold all kinds of liniments with much public commotion" and continued to use various cures in public places as well as at his inn, the "Blaue Hand" at the hay market.[72] When they confronted him, he just laughed at them and replied that "he was not a 'chyrurgus' but a 'medicus'" which almost led to a brawl with the enraged surgeons. While some of the doctors designated as "quacks" had in fact been to medical school and therefore felt they were superior to some of the resident healers, especially as they had travelled far and gained a lot of experience, there were also those among them who knew little about (Galenic) medicine but were well versed in early modern "pharmaceutical advertising".[73]

Summary

Let us summarize the differences between medical pluralism prior to 1800 and its present manifestations. The following description by historian Barbara Duden applies to the past: "The real and symbolic complexity of the physical

---

69   Hörnigk (1638), p. 172.
70   See, for instance, Jütte (2001); Katritzky (2007).
71   HAStK, Zunft-Akten 357, f. 12r (5.2.1614).
72   HAStK, Zunft-Akten 379, p. 245 (17.5.1649).
73   Cf. Zimmermann (1968), pp. 49ff.

body finds reflection in the complexity of the social community of healers or of those offering practical medical help."[74] This kind of medical pluralism is ubiquitous in pre-modern sources. Investigation into the professionalization of the medical system shows that the transition from professional pluralism to the domination of experts only proceeded gradually since the late eighteenth and early nineteenth centuries.[75] The extensive competences of modern physicians in the realm of scientific diagnosis and therapy are fully legitimized by their successful university education and supported by society. The numerous specialities within technical-scientific medicine are guided by the idea of the body as a biochemical organism. It is a school of thought that regards disease as a spatially localizable disorder, a kind of functional disturbance that can be corrected by using specific surgical and pharmaceutical interventions. Physicians play the part of technical specialists to whom patients, as ignorant laypersons, entrust their organism to be repaired in accordance with the ideology of the medical-industrial complex.

While today's system of specialization is informed by developments within the various disciplines and refers to scientific progress and insights, the specialization known in late mediaeval and early modern society did not rely on formal training and not even on academic attainment. Unlike today it was in those days not a matter of finding one's way around a complex medical hierarchy with the help of an academic physician, thus achieving a cure, but of finding, with the help of a lay system, the right specialist for a particular cause of disease. Outside the established healing community (physicians, surgeons, apothecaries) existed dozens of providers of unconventional but nevertheless specific health-care services, from executioners and wise women to miracle healers specialized in blessings and the laying-on of hands.

If one fell ill in early modern times one had access to a considerable array of healers even if one was not well off. There were non-official or half-official specialists for all the more or less clearly defined afflictions: cutters of hernias, tooth pullers for toothaches, bonesetters (who usually also served as executioners) for dislocations, enchanters and wise women for lumbago. Research into the attitude to illness in early modern Bologna showed that patients chose their healers horizontally or vertically, guided by aspects of reciprocity or the search for protection or, in other words, according to a social logic that they themselves determined.[76]

Medical culture, usually interpreted as a hierarchy of forms of knowledge in medical history, is consequently based on the "cultural interpretation of the body".[77] But the term "medical pluralism" only applies with restrictions here. Prior to 1800, the healing system was neither homogeneous nor harmonious but riddled with conflict. We must nonetheless not base our description of these competing systems on the differentiations we make today between ra-

---

74 Duden (1987), p. 40.
75 Jütte (2003).
76 See Wolff (2003).
77 Duden (1987), p. 41.

tional and irrational, natural and supernatural, religious and superstitious, especially when referring to the period prior to 1850 when this kind of dichotomy was still largely incomprehensible.

Today we have a clear dividing line between professional and other healers that is strictly monitored by the legislator, for the "benefit" of the patient. Non-medical practitioners nowadays have to undergo training and pass examinations before the relevant authorities to obtain a licence. Traditional healing rituals, reaching from faith healing to the charming of warts, although they survived, have been marginalised.[78]

The process of professionalization that has penetrated the health care system since the eighteenth century at the latest also affected day-to-day medical culture. The lay system is no longer permitted to provide any services apart from nursing and care. Public health pioneers like Johann Peter Frank warned subjects not to combat any disease without directions from a physician. Since then an increasing part of the population has heeded this advice and consulted medical experts when they were ill, even if they were not always university trained physicians but often semi-professional healers. The social reasons for their behaviour are obvious. The degree of medicalization, or – more precisely – the density of physicians also played an important part in this. The change occurred as part of the overall modernization of society.

In early modern times the old pluralism still prevailed in medicine. It was characterized by the lack of a monopoly and the openness of the system – at least from the point of view of the patient. Or, as Cologne councillor and lawyer Hermann Weinsberg (1508–1597) once wrote when he listed professions known to him in alphabetical order: "For 'Q' I could find only quack which I did not want to add since it was dealt with under physician."[79]

Bibliography

Ahrendt-Schulte, Ingrid: Weise Frauen – böse Weiber: die Geschichte der Frauen in der Frühen Neuzeit. Freiburg/Brsg. 1994.

Blankenburg, Susann: Das Hebammenwesen Augsburgs zur Zeit der Reichsstadt unter besonderer Berücksichtigung der Hebammenordnungen. Diss. Universität Ulm 2003.

Böhme, Gernot: Wissenschaftliches und lebensweltliches Wissen am Beispiel der Verwissenschaftlichung der Geburtshilfe. In: Stehr, Nico; Meja, Volker (eds.): Wissenssoziologie. Opladen 1981, pp. 445–463.

Boventer, Karl: Zur Medizingeschichte im Bereich des Regierungsbezirks Aachen bis zur Mitte des 19. Jahrhunderts. In: Zeitschrift des Aachener Geschichtsvereins 83 (1976), pp. 59–141.

Bühring, Martina: Heiler und Heilen: eine medizinhistorische und methodologische Studie über Handauflegen und Besprechen in Berlin. Berlin 1993.

Bullough, Vern: The development of medicine as profession. Basel; New York 1966.

Chmielewski-Hagius, Anita: "Was ich greif, das weich ...": Heilerwesen in Oberschwaben. Münster 1996.

---

78 See, for example, Bühring (1993); Chmielewski-Hagius (1996).
79 Weinsberg (1926), p. 188.

Cipolla, Carlo M.: Cristofano and the plague: a study in the history of public health in the age of Galileo. London 1973.

Diepgen, Paul: Volksmedizin und wissenschaftliche Heilkunde. Ihre geschichtlichen Beziehungen (1937). In: Grabner, Elfriede (ed.): Volksmedizin. Probleme und Forschungsgeschichte. Darmstadt 1967, pp. 200–222.

Dinges, Martin: Süd-Nord-Gefälle in der Pestbekämpfung. Italien, Deutschland und England im Vergleich. In: Eckart, Wolfgang U.; Jütte, Robert (eds.): Das europäische Gesundheitssystem. Gemeinsamkeiten und Unterschiede in historischer Perspektive. Stuttgart 1994, pp. 19–51.

Dinges, Martin: Pest und Staat. Von der Institutionengeschichte zur sozialen Konstruktion? In: Dinges, Martin; Schlich, Thomas (eds.): Neue Wege in der Seuchengeschichte. Stuttgart 1995, pp. 71–103.

Dinges, Martin: "Medicinische Policey" zwischen Heilkundigen und "Patienten" (1750–1830). In: Härter, Karl (ed.): Policey und frühneuzeitliche Gesellschaft. Frankfurt/Main 2000, pp. 263–295.

Dinges, Martin; Jütte, Robert (eds.): The transmission of health practices (c. 1500 to 2000). Stuttgart 2011.

Dornheim, Jutta: Selbsthilfegruppen und Gruppenselbsthilfe – Aspekte der Veränderung medikaler Alltagskultur. In: Jahrbuch des Instituts für Geschichte der Medizin der Robert Bosch Stiftung 5 (1986), pp. 7–33.

Dryander, Johannes: Practicierbüchlin außerlesener Artzeneystück [...]. Frankfurt/Main 1589.

Duden, Barbara: Geschichte unter der Haut. Ein Eisenacher Arzt und seine Patientinnen um 1730. Stuttgart 1987.

Eckardt, Stefan: Das Medizinalwesen der Reichsstadt Windsheim unter besonderer Berücksichtigung der Medizinal- und Badeordnungen. Diss. Universität Ulm 1991.

Elkeles, Barbara: Medicus und Medicaster. Zum Konflikt zwischen akademischer und empirischer Medizin im 17. und frühen 18. Jahrhundert. In: Medizinhistorisches Journal 22 (1987), pp. 197–211.

Fedro von Rhodach, Georg: Verantwortung Ge. Fedronis von Rhodoch/ auf etlich unglimpff der Sophistischen Artzten und seiner Missgünner/ darundten viel gewaltige geheimnuß/ zu gemeinem nutz der warhafftigem Medicin offenbart werden. [no place] 1566.

Fischer, Alfons: Geschichte des deutschen Gesundheitswesens. 2 vols. Leipzig 1933.

Fischer, Wolfgang: Das Medizinalwesen der Reichsstadt Wangen im Allgäu unter besonderer Berücksichtigung der Baderordnungen und Bestallungsurkunden. Diss. Universität Ulm 1991.

Frevert, Ute: Krankheit als politisches Problem, 1770–1880: soziale Unterschichten in Preußen zwischen medizinischer Polizei und staatlicher Sozialversicherung. Göttingen 1984.

Friedrich, Christoph; Müller-Jahncke, Wolf-Dieter: Geschichte der Pharmazie. Vol. 2: Von der Frühen Neuzeit bis zur Gegenwart. Eschborn 2005.

Gabler, Susanne: Das Hebammenwesen im Nördlingen des 16. Jahrhunderts. Diss. TU München 1985.

Gensthaler, Gerhard: Das Medizinalwesen der freien Reichsstadt Augsburg bis zum 16. Jahrhundert: mit Berücksichtigung der ersten Pharmakopö von 1564 und ihrer weiteren Ausgaben. Augsburg 1973.

Gossmann, Heinz: Das Collegium pharmaceuticum Norimbergense und sein Einfluß auf das Nürnbergische Medizinalwesen. Frankfurt/Main 1966.

Grell, Ole Peter; Cunningham, Andrew (eds.): Medicine and Religion in Enlightenment Europe. Aldershot 2007.

Groß, Dominik: Die Aufhebung des Wundarztberufs: Ursachen, Begleitumstände und Auswirkungen am Beispiel des Königreichs Württemberg (1806–1918). Stuttgart 1999.

Hammond, Mitchell Love: The origins of civic health care in early modern Germany. Blacksburg, VA 2000.

Hampp, Irmgard: Beschwörung, Segen, Gebet: Untersuchungen zum Zauberspruch aus dem Bereich der Volksheilkunde. Stuttgart 1961.

Hauri, Dieter (ed.): Die Steinschneider: eine Kulturgeschichte menschlichen Leidens und ärztlicher Kunst. Berlin 2010.

Heinemann, Franz: Die Henker und Scharfrichter als Volks- und Viehärzte seit dem Ausgang des Mittelalters. In: Schweizerisches Archiv für Volkskunde 4 (1900), pp. 1–16.

Herborn, Wolfgang: Der graduierte Ratsherr. Zur Entwicklung einer neuen Elite im Kölner Rat der frühen Neuzeit. In: Schilling, Heinz; Diederiks, Herman (eds.): Bürgerliche Eliten in den Niederlanden und in Nordwestdeutschland. Köln; Wien 1985, pp. 337–400.

Hieke, Karl: Der Landarzt und Arzneimittelfabrikant Johann Andreas Eisenbarth (1663–1727). Dargestellt anhand seiner Werbemittel und anderer zeitgenössischer Quellen. Sprockhövel 2002.

Horn, Sonia; Dorffner, Gabriele; Eichinger, Rosemarie (eds.): Wissensaustausch in der Medizin des 15. bis 18. Jahrhunderts. Wien 2007.

Hörnigk, Ludwig von: Politia medica [...]. Frankfurt/Main 1638.

Horst, Jakob: Ein Vorwarnung der Krancken vor ihrem selbs eigenen Schaden und vorseumnuß [...]. Görlitz 1574.

Hortzitz, Nicoline: Der "Judenarzt". Historische und sprachliche Untersuchungen zur Diskriminierung eines Berufsstands in der frühen Neuzeit. Heidelberg 1994.

Jäck, Karl; Nauck, Ernst Theodor: Zur Geschichte des Sanitätswesens im Fürstentum Fürstenberg. Allensbach/Bodensee 1951.

Jütte, Robert: Obrigkeitliche Armenfürsorge in deutschen Reichsstädten der frühen Neuzeit. Städtisches Armenwesen in Frankfurt am Main und Köln. Köln; Wien 1984.

Jütte, Robert: Patient und Heiler in der vorindustriellen Gesellschaft. Krankheits- und Gesundheitsverhalten im frühneuzeitlichen Köln. Habil. Fakultät für Geschichtswissenschaft und Philosophie, Universität Bielefeld 1989.

Jütte, Robert: Ärzte, Heiler und Patienten: medizinischer Alltag in der frühen Neuzeit. München; Zürich 1991.

Jütte, Robert: Bader, Barbiere und Hebammen. Heilkundige als Randgruppe? In: Hergemöller, Bernd-Ulrich (ed.): Randgruppen der spätmittelalterlichen Gesellschaft. 2nd revised ed. Warendorf 1995, pp. 89–120.

Jütte, Robert: Geschichte der Alternativen Medizin. München 1996.

Jütte, Robert: Zur Funktion und sozialen Stellung jüdischer "gelehrter" Ärzte im spätmittelalterlichen und frühneuzeitlichen Deutschland. In: Schwinges, Rainer C. (ed.): Gelehrte im Alten Reich. Zur Sozial- und Wirkungsgeschichte akademischer Eliten des 14. bis 16. Jahrhundert. Berlin 1996, pp. 159–179.

Jütte, Robert (ed.): The Doctor on the Stage: performing and curing in early modern Europe. (=special issue of Ludica. Annali di storia e civiltà del gioco 5/6 (2000)). Roma 2001.

Jütte, Robert: La professione medica. In: Storia della Scienca. Enciclopedia Italiana Treccani. Vol. 7. Roma 2003, pp. 862–863.

Jütte, Robert: Gesundheitsverständnis im Zeitalter (un-)begrenzter medizinischer Möglichkeiten. In: Schäfer, Daniel et al. (eds.): Gesundheitskonzepte im Wandel. Geschichte, Ethik und Gesellschaft. Stuttgart 2008, pp. 53–62.

Jütte, Robert: Menschliche Gewebe und Organe als Bestandteil einer rationalen Medizin im 18. Jahrhundert. In: Helm, Jürgen; Wilson, Renate (eds.): Medical Theory and Therapeutic Practice in the Eighteenth Century. A Transatlantic Perspective. Stuttgart 2008, pp. 137–158.

Katritzky, Margaret Agnes: Women, medicine, and theatre, 1500–1750: literary mountebanks and performing quacks. Aldershot, Hants et al. 2007.

Keussen, Hermann: Die alte Universität Köln. Grundzüge ihrer Verfassung und Geschichte. Köln 1934.

Kintzinger, Martin: Status medicorum. Mediziner in der städtischen Gesellschaft des 14. bis 17. Jahrhunderts. In: Johanek, Peter (ed.): Städtisches Gesundheits- und Fürsorgewesen vor 1800. Köln; Wien; Weimar 2000, pp. 63–93.

Kinzelbach, Annemarie: Gesundbleiben, Krankwerden, Armsein in der frühneuzeitlichen Gesellschaft: Gesunde und Kranke in den Reichsstädten Überlingen und Ulm, 1500–1700. Stuttgart 1995.

Kleinman, Arthur: Patients and healers in the context of culture. An exploration of the borderland between anthropology, medicine and psychiatry. Berkeley; London 1980.

Klimpel, Volker: Das Dresdner Collegium Medico-Chirurgicum. Frankfurt/Main 1995.

Knefelkamp, Ulrich: Das Gesundheits- und Fürsorgewesen der Stadt Freiburg im Breisgau im Mittelalter. Freiburg/Brsg. 1981.

Krauß, Martin: Armenwesen und Gesundheitsfürsorge in Mannheim vor der Industrialisierung: 1750–1850/60. Sigmaringen 1993.

Lindemann, Mary: Health & healing in eighteenth-century Germany. Baltimore, MD 1996.

Loetz, Francisca: Vom Kranken zum Patienten: "Medikalisierung" und medizinische Vergesellschaftung am Beispiel Badens 1750–1850. Stuttgart 1993.

Loytved, Christine (ed.): Von der Wehemutter zur Hebamme: die Gründung von Hebammenschulen mit Blick auf ihren politischen Stellenwert und praktischen Nutzen. Osnabrück 2001.

MacLean, Ian: Logic, signs, and nature in the Renaissance: the case of learned medicine. Cambridge 2002.

Mering, Friedrich E. von: Die Pest in Cöln im Jahre 1665–1666. In: Annalen des Historischen Vereins für den Niederrhein 6 (1857), pp. 137–157.

Möller, Caren: Medizinalpolizei: die Theorie des staatlichen Gesundheitswesens im 18. und 19. Jahrhundert. Frankfurt/Main 2005.

Müller, Christina Beate Ingeborg: Das Medizinalwesen der Reichsstadt Isny im Allgäu vom ausgehenden Mittelalter bis zum Ende der reichstädtischen Zeit. Diss. Universität Ulm 1994.

Müller-Jahncke, Wolf-Dieter: Astrologisch-magische Theorie und Praxis in der Heilkunde der frühen Neuzeit. Wiesbaden et al. 1985.

Münch, Ragnhild: Gesundheitswesen im 18. und 19. Jahrhundert: das Berliner Beispiel. Berlin 1995.

Münkle, Werner: Das Medizinalwesen der Reichsstadt Hall vom ausgehenden Mittelalter bis zum Ende der reichstädtischen Zeit: eine Auswertung der Bader-, Barbier- und Medizinalordnungen. Diss. Universität Ulm 1992.

Neubrand, Robert: Das Medizinalwesen der Reichsstadt Ravensburg unter besonderer Berücksichtigung der Stadtphysici, Bader und Barbiere: vom ausgehenden Mittelalter bis zum Ende der Reichsstadtzeit. Diss. Universität Ulm 1994.

Neumann, Josef N.: "…davon künfftig auch andere Curen Nutzen haben können" – Körperkonzept, anatomisches Wissen, medizinische Praxis in der Frühneuzeit bis Ende des 18. Jahrhunderts. In: Schultka, Rüdiger; Neumann, Josef N. (eds.): Anatomie und anatomische Sammlungen im 18. Jahrhundert. Anlässlich der 250. Wiederkehr des Geburtstages von Philipp Friedrich Theodor Meckel (1755–1803). Berlin 2007, pp. 73–95.

Nowosadtko, Jutta: Wer Leben nimmt, kann auch Leben geben: Scharfrichter und Wasenmeister als Heilkundige in der Frühen Neuzeit. In: Medizin, Gesellschaft und Geschichte 12 (1994), pp. 43–74.

O'Neill, Mary R.: Sacerdote ovvero strione: Ecclesiastical and Superstitious Remedies in 16th Century Italy. In: Kaplan, Steven L. (ed.): Understanding Popular Culture. Berlin; New York; Amsterdam 1984, pp. 53–83.

Pelling, Margaret: Appearances and Reality: Barber-surgeons, the Body and Disease. In: Beier, A. L.; Finlay, Roger (eds.): London 1500–1700: The Making of the Metropolis. London; New York 1986, pp. 82–112.

Pies, Eike: Eisenbarth: das Ende einer Legende. Leben und Wirken des genialen Chirurgen, weit gereisten Landarztes und ersten deutschen Arzneimittelfabrikanten Johann Andreas Eisenbarth (1663–1727). Wuppertal 2004.

Plank, Thomas: Das Medizinalwesen der Reichsstadt Regensburg unter Berücksichtigung des Bader-, Barbier- und Wundarztwesens vom Beginn des 14. Jahrhunderts bis 1803. Diss. Universität Ulm 1999.

Remmen, Hans: Die Beziehungen des Fabricius Hildanus zu Köln an Hand seiner Observationes et Curationes. Hilden 1965.

Risse, Guenter: Epidemics and Medicine. The influence of disease on medical practice and thought. In: Bulletin of the History of Medicine 53 (1979), pp. 505–519.

Rosen, George: From Medical Police to social medicine. Essays on the history of health care. New York 1974.

Rummel, Walter: Weise Frauen und weise Männer im Kampf gegen Hexerei. Die Widerlegung einer modernen Fabel. In: Dipper, Christof; Klinkhammer, Lutz; Nützenadel, Alexander (eds.): Europäische Sozialgeschichte. Festschrift für Wolfgang Schieder. Berlin 2000, pp. 353–376.

Sander, Sabine: Handwerkschirurgen: Sozialgeschichte einer verdrängten Berufsgruppe. Göttingen 1989.

Schaffer, Wolfgang; Werner, Wolfgang F. (eds.): Rheinische Wehemütter: 200 Jahre Ausbildung, Professionalisierung, Disziplinierung von Hebammen. Begleitband zur Ausstellung. Essen 2009.

Schenda, Rudolf: Der "gemeine Mann" und sein medikales Verhalten im 16. und 17. Jahrhundert. In: Telle, Joachim (ed.): Pharmazie und der gemeine Mann. Wolfenbüttel 1982, pp. 9–20.

Schilling, Heinz: Religion und Gesellschaft in der calvinistischen Republik der Vereinigten Niederlande – "Öffentlichkeitskirche" und Säkularisation; Ehe und Hebammenwesen; Presbyterien und politische Partizipation. In: Petri, Franz (ed.): Kirche und gesellschaftlicher Wandel in deutschen und niederländischen Städten der werdenden Neuzeit. Köln; Wien 1980, pp. 197–250.

Schipperges, Heinrich: Motivation und Legitimation des ärztlichen Handelns. In: Schipperges, Heinrich; Seidler, Eduard; Unschuld, Paul U. (eds.): Krankheit, Heilkunst, Heilung. Freiburg/Brsg.; München 1978, pp. 447–489.

Schmidt, Alfred: Die Kölner Apotheken: von der ältesten Zeit bis zum Ende der reichsstädtischen Verfassung. 2nd, enlarged and improved ed. Köln 1931.

Schwanitz, Hedwig: Krankheit – Armut – Alter: Gesundheitsfürsorge und Medizinalwesen in Münster während des 19. Jahrhunderts. Münster 1990.

Schwartz, Friedrich Wilhelm: Idee und Konzeption der frühen territorialstaatlichen Gesundheitspflege in Deutschland ("Medizinische Polizei") in der ärztlichen und staatswissenschaftlichen Fachliteratur des 16.–18. Jahrhunderts. Frankfurt/Main 1973.

Seidel, Hans-Christoph: Eine neue "Kultur des Gebärens": die Medikalisierung von Geburt im 18. und 19. Jahrhundert in Deutschland. Stuttgart 1998.

Seidler, Eduard: Primärerfahrung von Not und Hilfe. In: Schipperges, Heinrich; Seidler, Eduard; Unschuld, Paul U. (eds.): Krankheit, Heilkunst, Heilung. Freiburg/Brsg.; München 1978, pp. 399–418.

Signori, Gabriela: Wunder: eine historische Einführung. Frankfurt/Main et al. 2007.

Stadlober-Degwerth, Marion: (Un)Heimliche Niederkunften: Geburtshilfe zwischen Hebammenkunst und medizinischer Wissenschaft. Köln et al. 2008.

Steinhilber, Wilhelm: Das Gesundheitswesen im alten Heilbronn 1281–1871. Heilbronn 1956.

Stenzel, Oliver: Medikale Differenzierung. Der Konflikt zwischen akademischer Medizin und Laienheilkunde im 18. Jahrhundert. Heidelberg 2005.

Stuart, Kathy: Defiled trades and social outcasts: honor and ritual pollution in early modern Germany. Cambridge 1999.

Terhalle, Hermann: Das Kurmainzer Medizinalwesen vom Spätmittelalter bis zum Ende des 18. Jahrhunderts. Mainz 1965.

Thomas, Keith: Religion and the decline of magic. Studies in popular belief in sixteenth and seventeenth century England. Harmondsworth 1988.

Treue, Wilhelm: Mit den Augen ihrer Leibärzte. Düsseldorf 1955.

Wahrig, Bettina; Sohn, Werner (eds.): Zwischen Aufklärung, Policey und Verwaltung. Zur Genese des Medizinalwesens 1750–1850. Wiesbaden 2003.

Walter, Tilmann: Ärztehaushalte im 16. Jahrhundert. Einkünfte, Status und Praktiken der Repräsentation. In: Medizin, Gesellschaft und Geschichte 27 (2008), pp. 31–73.

Watermann, Rembert Antonius: Vom Medizinalwesen des Kurfürstentums Köln und der Reichsstadt Köln (1761–1802). Neuss 1977.

Weingärtner, Elke: Das Medizinal- und Fürsorgewesen der Stadt Trier im Mittelalter und der frühen Neuzeit. Diss. Universität Mainz 1981.

Weinsberg, Hermann: Das Buch Weinsberg: Kölner Denkwürdigkeiten aus dem 16. Jahrhundert. Vol. 5, ed. by Josef Stein. Bonn 1926.

Wiesner, Merry: Working Women in Renaissance Germany. New Brunswick, NJ 1986.

Wischhöfer, Bettina: Krankheit, Gesundheit und Gesellschaft in der Aufklärung: das Beispiel Lippe 1750–1830. Frankfurt/Main 1991.

Witzel, Alexander (ed.): Ein Lesebuch zur Unterhaltung und Belehrung für Ärzte. Stuttgart 1990.

Wolff, Eberhard: Medikalisierung von unten? Das Beispiel der jüdischen Krankenbesuchsgesellschaften. In: Wahrig, Bettina; Sohn, Werner (eds.): Zwischen Aufklärung, Policey und Verwaltung. Zur Genese des Medizinalwesens 1750–1850. Wiesbaden 2003, pp. 179–190.

Zimmermann, Heinz: Arzneimittelwerbung in Deutschland vom Beginn des 16. Jahrhunderts bis zum Ende des 18. Jahrhunderts. Dargestellt vorzugsweise an Hand von Archivalien der Freien Reichs-, Handels- und Messestadt Frankfurt am Main. Diss. Universität Marburg 1968.

Medical Pluralism and the Medical Marketplace in Early Modern Italy

David Gentilcore

I am writing this contribution in the land of the medical marketplace. I am not referring here to proposals by prime minister David Cameron and his Conservative Party for the reform of the UK's National Health Service, only the latest in a long series of such reforms along market-orientated lines (or to 'bring in' the market). Rather, I am referring to the medical marketplace used as a model for the understanding of healing provision and healing strategies in the past. In this chapter I would like to compare the use of the marketplace model with that of the pluralism model by historians, especially as it concerns what English-speaking historians refer to as the 'early modern' period: 1500–1800 (although the chronological parameters can vary according to what is being studied).

The use of the marketplace model has a history of its own, beginning in the 1980s on into the present day, primarily as a way of conveying 'the pluralistic diversity of medical provision' in early modern England, to quote from a recent volume devoted to it, edited by Mark Jenner and Patrick Wallis.[1] The model carried all before it, quickly becoming 'part of the vernacular of early modern English history', at a time when the social history of medicine and the 'view from below' were just establishing themselves.[2]

There is no denying that the marketplace model was then a breath of fresh air. Previously, if early modern history of medicine had strayed into the area of medical practice at all (something it rarely did), it was to focus on the notional tripartite occupational hierarchy of physician-surgeon-apothecary; other healers were either ignored or labelled 'quacks'. The medical marketplace model, by contrast, offered a new vision of (and approach towards) the past: one that was diverse, pluralistic, pre-professional and commercialised, in which patients were active and promiscuous. It looked to social and economic history and made use of a broader range of sources. So convincing and pervasive was the model that it was used to describe medical provision not just in early modern England, but in times and places as diverse as the Graeco-Roman world, Renaissance Florence and nineteenth-century South Africa.[3]

At its most convincing, the marketplace model might be used to describe a particular stage in the process of the commercialisation of health care. Harold Cook used it this way when he suggested 'the creation of a market for medical skills and services' which, by the end of the seventeenth century, had

---

1 Jenner/Wallis (2007), p. 4.
2 Jenner/Wallis (2007), p. 3.
3 Jenner/Wallis (2007), pp. 1 and 2: referring to Nutton (1992), Park (1985), and Deacon (2004).

overtaken the London College of Physicians' attempts at regulation.[4] The usage offered a specific chronology and a strong relationship to other historical literature. Cook also used the expression in a more generalised way, to convey the variety of sources of medical therapy. This second use of the marketplace model, which would predominate amongst historians, is the much less convincing one. Used in this way, the model became 'little more than a descriptive commonplace', giving little indication of what factors determined the structures involved and the shifting relations between them.[5]

Jenner and Wallis point out that the model's weakness derives from 'the lack of a single clear definition of the "marketplace"' by historians; they suggest, as a solution, 'a more rigorous engagement with what is meant by the medical marketplace' in their explorations of 'the economy of health and medicine'.[6]

The marketplace model is, as its name suggests, an economic one. This is both its strength and its weakness. It sits well within a prevalent idea of medical services as commodities to be bought and sold, where the patient is first and foremost a consumer.[7] In the case of the marketplace, the patient is able to exercise a degree of choice amongst the various services provided, which are in competition with one another. It is less useful in explaining pluralistic medical environments. Here, we must be careful what we mean by 'pluralism'. In the literature regarding early modern England, plurality is usually shorthand for variety: for a medical spectrum going from domestic medicine to professional physicians. If they occupy the same marketplace, it is because they belong to the same medical system, at the most representing different ends of that system. By way of example, this is what John Henry has written about popular healers in early modern England: 'the wise men and wise women called upon by the villagers, as far as we can tell, held to roughly the same set of beliefs about humoural pathology, and used the same kind of treatments, herbal remedies and manipulations as any physician or surgeon'.[8]

But what about where archival and printed sources give us a picture of popular medicine that is qualitatively different from canonical medicine, with radically different explanatory models? What happens when popular healing is on a different spectrum altogether? The plurality of different therapeutic forms I felt best suited my findings for early modern southern Italy was a long way from Henry's notion of 'plurality'.

By way of example, let us consider the following illness episode, one of many similar recounted in Italian archival records. When confronted with the inevitable reality of disease, how did the people of early modern Italy react? Of the different forms of healing available, what factors determined which ones they turned to?

4   Cook (1986), pp. 28–69.
5   Jenner/Wallis (2007), p. 6.
6   Jenner/Wallis (2007), p. 7.
7   Han (2002), paragraph 6.2.
8   Henry (1991), p. 203.

In June of 1704, in the town of Oria (southern Apulia), Antonia Jurlaro recounted how her daughter Domenica had become 'gravely ill' with severe pains in her genitalia, accompanied by high fever. Antonia fetched the town's municipal doctor who examined and treated the girl, but without any improvement in her condition. Domenica was also bled three times by a surgeon, Simone Papatodero. Several days later Antonia was washing clothes at one of the town wells, despairing of her daughter's health. A woman named Onofria Bufalo overheard her and said it was like an illness she had suffered for a whole year. Onofria added that she might be able to get her the same remedy she had taken. Such was Antonia's anxiety that, she recounted, 'having heard this it seemed to take me a thousand years to finish washing the clothes'. Antonia immediately went to Onofria's house and beseeched her to give her the remedy.

At this point Antonia's account takes an unexpected twist. Onofria, who had a local reputation as a magical healer, or *magara*, went to examine Domenica. Onofria identified it as the same affliction and said she would go to the surgeon Papatodero for the remedy, though he did not give it to everyone. She warned Antonia not to tell anyone about it.

The next morning Onofria told Antonia that she had been unable to find Papatodero and so would have to go to the nearby town of Francavilla for the remedy. She asked for seven *carlini* and five *grana* in payment. This was a substantial sum: what a peasant labourer might receive for three or four days' work. Later, Onofria gave Domenica some of the remedy with honey, and prepared an enema of rue and sage which she administered – acting like a physician, surgeon and apothecary combined. Domenica slept the whole night through and seemed better the next day.

However, at this point some kind of disagreement ensued between Antonia and Onofria. Onofria shouted that Antonia and her daughter should be grateful for what she had done. Domenica's condition began to worsen. Onofria said she required more medicine, which Antonia said she could not afford. Onofria offered to take something as a pledge if Antonia could not scrape the money together. But friends of Antonia's were becoming suspicious and advised her to stay away from the 'vile Onofria' and instead place her daughter's health in God's hands. Domenica's condition continued to get worse. Such was the stinging pain in her genitals 'as if there was a sea urchin in there'.

Mother and daughter became convinced that Onofria had put a spell on Domenica. Magical healers like Onofria were reputed to know how to harm as well as heal, especially in view of the fact that Domenica had had a row with Onofria the previous May. They were both part of a group of women out gleaning barley when Onofria had the idea of hiding one of the sacks. The other women agreed and did so, despite Domenica's opposition. When the estate factor found the hidden bag, the women blamed Domenica. Later, Domenica recalled Onofria's words to her: 'I'll make you sorry for this and I'll be damned if I won't put a spell on you that will have you chewing your fingernails'. With this event in mind, Antonia and Domenica then decided to go and

see their parish priest to heal the spell. He gave Domenica a blessing and advised them to denounce Onofria to the bishop for 'superstitious acts'. The
surgeon Papatodero suggested the same course of action, 'since we are the
doctors and not her'.

The resulting deposition before the episcopal tribunal in Oria is the only
reason the illness episode has come down to us. Yet it introduces many aspects
of early modern medical pluralism, outlining as it did Antonia's strategies in
searching for a cure for her daughter's illness, the causation of which she diagnosed first as natural and then as supernatural. In this therapeutic calculus, the
availability of medical practitioners was certainly one factor considered; but
we must also bear in mind others as diverse as the cost of the healer's services
and treatment, their reputation, their suitability to the disease in question and
its underlying causation, as well as the past experience of the sick themselves,
their family and friends.

The model I proposed for my 1998 book 'Healers and Healing in Early
Modern Italy' was one of three concentric and permeable rings, in the form of
a Venn diagram, labelled 'medical', 'ecclesiastical' and 'popular', respectively.[9] The rings refer both to the types of healers and sources of healing, and to
aetiological categories. As a model, I hoped it would allow us to give due attention to the attitudes and actions of both healers and the sick. The model is
admittedly anthropological; but it does allow for historical change. Indeed,
the circles are continually shifting in relation to one another, as are the places
of individual healers and sources of healing. People did not belong or limit
themselves uniquely to a single sphere – churchmen to the ecclesiastical, physicians to the medical and peasants and the urban poor to the popular. After
all, in early modern Italy popes depended on their own private physicians and
surgeons; physicians could find themselves the victims of sorcery or the ben-
eficiaries of miracles; and the poor could make use of the services of community practitioners free of charge. In other words, people moved from one
sphere to another according to circumstance and need. As a model, I thought
it best captured the findings of my own research.

My medical pluralism model was indebted to the work of Jean-Pierre
Goubert, who proposed the co-existence of three different cultural strata in the
early modern period, each of which had its origins in a different 'age'. (Not a
Venn diagram but a palimpsest.) During what Goubert labelled the 'cosmo-
logical age', illness was regarded as a rupture of the order of the world. Its
therapeutic was likewise of a sacred order, expressed in a manner that was
both concrete and symbolic. The second age was that of 'dominant Christian-
ity', which linked illness to evil and stressed the salvation of the soul over the
death of the body. Finally, the 'modern age', beginning with Renaissance hu-
manism, secularized the things of body and nature. Illness arose from a natural disorder, which human knowledge and 'science' were capable of compre-
hending. Eventually, the medical 'professionals' drove out the sorcerers, saints

9   Gentilcore (1998), p. 3.

and healers. For Goubert, the goal of research was 'the analysis of these three cultural "strata", the study of their antagonisms and their interactions, even their recovery and their condemnation by the third stratum at the end of the eighteenth century'.[10]

Whilst keeping Goubert's schema in mind, my own emphasis on the sufferer's point of view led me to prefer the more overtly anthropological approach first proposed by Arthur Kleinman in 1978. This posited the existence of three social 'arenas' within most health-care systems: popular, professional and folk.[11] Indeed, I wish I had paid more attention to Kleinman's model back in 1998; in particular, its emphasis on the popular arena, which was the largest and central circle in the diagram, containing the 'family context of sickness and care', wherein most sickness is managed, in both Western and non-Western societies. (By contrast, my overlapping rings had all been the same size.) Aside from the model's form, what most appealed to me was Kleinman's view of health care and illness as a cultural system. Each of the arenas in Kleinman's model were culturally constructed, in the sense that each offered its own explanatory models for illness episodes, shared by sufferers, family members and practitioners. Exploration of these explanatory models should focus 'on actual transactions between patients (and their families) and practitioners', Kleinman argued. In this way the investigator would be able to elicit 'the real structures of knowledge, logic, and relevance that operate in different health care sectors and systems, and [reveal] how they are *used* in the healing process'.[12]

How has the medical pluralism model fared? It has to be said that, like the marketplace model, it is sometimes reduced to the level of descriptive label: an affirmation of the co-existence of a variety of different healing forms and explanatory systems. I have in mind Elizabeth Whitaker's ethnography of medical pluralism in modern-day Emilia Romagna.[13] It may also say something about just how these forms co-exist or came to co-exist, as in Whitaker's case (in a layering that echoes Goubert's model).

Much the same can be said about the use of medical pluralism in Christos Papadopoulos's 2008 PhD thesis, supervised by Harold Cook and Andrew Wear. It was very gratifying indeed that this study of Greek medical culture in the eighteenth and early nineteenth century adopted my medical pluralism model as its guiding principle – changing only the labelling of the respective spheres: 'medical' to 'academic', 'ecclesiastical' to 'religious', and 'popular' to 'traditional'.[14] The content of the spheres was different, too, reflecting the different medical reality: medical authority was both Greek and Venetian in influence, religious forms took in both Greek Orthodox and Muslim, whilst 'traditional' practices were arguably more similar to what I had found in southern

10   Goubert (1987), p. 54.
11   Kleinman (1978), pp. 86–87.
12   Kleinman (1978), pp. 87, 89. Emphasis in original.
13   Whitaker (2003). Here, the forms are humoural, biomedical and personalistic/spiritual.
14   Papadopoulos (2008), p. 24.

Italy. The thesis is particularly strong on presenting and analysing everyday lived experience. Disease and responses to it are explored as theory, learning, tradition and belief; but also as practice. Whilst all of this was slow to change, just as the Greek world itself was slow to change during the period under study, the thesis explores shifts where they did occur, especially in terms of medical knowledge and the public roles of physicians. The thesis has weaknesses. Whilst it is rich in data and description concerning the Greek medical world, the use of the medical pluralism model is not so much analytical as descriptive.

More critical in approach was Alexandra Bamji's 2007 PhD thesis on religion and disease in seventeenth-century Venice, supervised by Mary Laven. Bamji declared that my medical pluralism model also applied there. What she drew from the model was 'the recourse to multiple practitioners' it elucidated.[15] Given this focus, it is not entirely surprising that she then sought 'to reconfigure the model of "medical pluralism" by revealing both the diversity of any given practitioner's activity, and the complex composition of individual remedies'.[16] This was certainly a worthwhile adjunct, particularly its detailed discussion of the pluralistic activities of female healers in Venice. Bamji did not limit herself to the pluralism model, but drew on the medical marketplace model as well, which she felt useful in highlighting the issue of patient choice and the patient-practitioner encounter as an exchange. Bamji clearly delineated the relative merits and limitations of the two models.[17] Although this came at the price of oversimplifying both of them, her work drew attention to the fact that both models had (and have) their different uses, even if these are difficult to tease apart. This is something I have also tried to grapple with. And though I remain attached to the pluralism model, I too have had recourse to the market in particular instances (which I shall return to shortly); but in the case of early modern Italy, it is a 'regulated marketplace', given the active role of the various medical authorities, as opposed to the supposedly free English market.[18]

And grapple with it we must. There is an unfortunate tendency to use the expressions 'medical pluralism' and 'medical marketplace' interchangeably.[19] Using the terms interchangeably suggests we are back to simple labels about the variety of medical provision. But a model should do more than that. For a model to be useful, it must account for decisions made by the sick and their

15   Bamji (2007), pp. 11, 55.
16   Bamji (2007), p. 20.
17   Bamji (2007), pp. 232–234.
18   Gentilcore (2005).
19   This occurs, just by way of example, in María Luz López Terrada's discussion of the therapeutic forms practised in sixteenth-century Valencia. López Terrada (2007), p. 9. But it is possible to distinguish. In this case, although this is never made explicit in the article, it would seem that when medical professionals, like the university elite, sought to exercise control over the medical field, the expression marketplace is more useful. Whereas, when the medical field is explored from the point of view of its use by sick themselves, then pluralism might be the more relevant concept.

carers. It must account for which healing therapies/strategies are undertaken in which circumstances.

To illustrate the relative strengths and weaknesses, or better yet, the appropriateness of the two respective models, I would like to conclude by discussing two 'test cases' deriving from my own research: tarantism and charlatanism.

Found in southern Apulia, tarantism was a structured and ritualised response to deep psychological malaise, which included the evocation and discharge of the crisis by traditional forms of music and dance.[20] The typical case scenario was that of a man or woman falling into a deep depression, triggered by some social occurrence with which the individual cannot cope, but identified in this culture as being caused by the bite of the tarantula spider. Once the malady was thus identified, the sufferer proceeded to the only remedy regarded as efficacious: that of the dance, and the ritual paraphernalia associated with it, which continued publicly for days on end, till the sufferer pronounced himself cured. The dances were repeated every year on the anniversary of the 'bite'. Medical anthropologists of the present use the expression 'culture-bound disorder' to explain such maladies.

The Spanish American malady known as *susto* ('fright' or 'shock') is an analogous form of behavioural syndrome, by which its victims seek 'to correct troublesome social relations or to call attention to their social or emotional needs'.[21] The Taiwanese disorder known as *ching* (which also translates as 'fright') is another example. In the context of a study on *ching*, Arthur Kleinman defines culture-bound disorders as 'illnesses associated with culturally unique patterns of meaning superimposed on diseases that are universal'.[22] Such cultural patterning is particularly evident for such things as depression, anxiety neurosis and other ubiquitous psychiatric diseases. The healing of the illness within such a cultural system is often the management of the underlying disease, rather than its cure. Such would seem to be the case with tarantism, especially if we consider the *rimorso*, the annual repetition of the symptoms and dancing. For the society concerned, the important thing is that the ritual be perceived to treat the malady. Indeed, because indigenous healing is part of the same cultural system as the illness, it must heal; just as other medical forms, such as modern professional clinical care, must fail to heal.[23]

Thus only the traditional ritual elements could heal a *tarantato*, labelled as such by the victim and those around him. The particular efficacy of the ritual was recognised by local physicians like Epifanio Ferdinando (1621) and Niccolò Caputi (1741) who each explained this efficacy according to the science of their day.[24] Closer to our own time, as research in the 1950s found, psychiatric treatment in hospital proved ineffective for those patients convinced that

---

20   The following discussion is based on Gentilcore (2000).
21   Rubel/O'Nell/Collado-Ardón (1984), p. 113.
22   Kleinman (1980), p. 77.
23   Kleinman (1980), pp. 362–363.
24   Gentilcore (2001).

they were *tarantati*. In the same way, remedies proposed in the early modern period by canonical medicine, the Church (canonical exorcisms), and even local cunning folk, were destined to fail, preparing the way for the ritual dance. The medical pluralism model is best suited to account for such an explanatory model of illness, and the behaviour associated with it. Economic calculations or relationships did not come into play, although the therapy could be quite a costly one.

My second test case concerns medical charlatans. By 'charlatans' I mean the several thousand sellers of medical remedies licensed by medical tribunals the length and breadth of the Italian peninsula to peddle and perform in public. In 'Healers and Healing' I used charlatans to illustrate the way the medical pluralism model could incorporate change: charlatans went from being quasi sacerdotal snake-charmers in the fifteenth century (the *sanpaolari*) to secular entrepreneurs selling famed patent remedies in the seventeenth (like the 'Orvietano', Girolamo Ferranti). In so doing, their place in the model shifted from one lying at the intersect of the popular and religious spheres to the intersect of the popular and medical spheres. However, what the pluralism model did not explain was the recourse to charlatans and the nature of transactions with them. So, when I came to explore this in 'Medical Charlatanism in Early Modern Italy' (2006), the marketplace model seemed much more useful.

Chapter seven, on 'commercial exchanges and therapeutic encounters', owes much to an economic view of the exchange, without (I hope) losing sight of its fundamentally cultural nature. The chapter looks first at the marketing and sale of medicines by charlatans, and second, the public response – how the remedies were purchased and used by the public. This, finally, lead me to look at the role some charlatans assumed as healers, treating the sick. Take the first of these. As exchanges of objects, for example, the selling and buying of charlatans' medicines were as much cultural events as examples of strictly economic behaviour. Italian charlatans spawned new entertainments to publicise and market their wares. As they began to develop novel products, like their electuaries and artificial balms, they had to encourage customers to attribute some meaning to them: hence their exaggerated claims. Not that these were new medicines in any absolute sense; the charlatans successfully combined the new with the familiar. On the one hand, they had to overcome, or at least placate, the hostility of vested medical interests in order to get licensed. They had to play within the rules, however negotiable, set by the physicians. On the other hand, charlatans' strategies were fully fledged commercial ventures which had to attract the public.

Charlatans made the most of their edge over apothecaries in not being constrained by guild policies and restrictions. They were more part of the 'informal' health sector, medically and commercially, apothecaries part of the 'formal' health sector: another model indebted to medical anthropology. Moreover, the charlatans' greatest presence on the medical scene, and the time when some of them at least made their greatest profits, both coincide with the continuing high prices of drugs as sold by apothecaries, relative to the cost of living. Charlatans moved in to fill the gap. They had to have a knowledge of the market.

Charlatans adopted various strategies to sell their wares. Pricing was one. Apothecaries had their prices set from year to year; charlatans, by contrast, were free to adopt a more flexible pricing policy, responsive to the most minute fluctuations. They could undercut apothecaries, their versions of theriac being a case in point. Charlatans sold cheaper imitations or variations rather than undercutting with like-for-like. They could also alter their prices to suit demand. However, it is worth stressing that the early modern marketplace was not a completely unfettered one. The authorities had a hand in setting charlatans' prices too. In setting prices for charlatans' wares, the officials took some account of the relative cost and number of ingredients used in their preparation, the cost of comparable medicines listed in the official pharmacopoeia, and their perceived usefulness, in a public health sense.

The medical authorities occasionally made explicit what was often implicit by attaching the proviso that the remedy be supplied free to the poor. The officials, in their paternalistic way, regarded certain simple medicines as useful and particularly suited to the poor. There were thus considerations of a moral nature too. Charlatans may have been entrepreneurs, operating in a competitive marketplace, but they were still affected by the dictates of the moral economy. Suffice it to say that there was little concept of the fixed price for any object or service. A range of considerations and mitigating circumstances came into play: personal, social, geographic, economic. Just as physicians would charge more for a home visit if it meant leaving the town gates, going out at night or treating a well-off patient, so charlatans varied their prices, mixing moral and market considerations.

As I hope this brief example of pricing illustrates, the marketplace model allowed me to conceptualise the nature of the market for the particular goods and services which Italian charlatans offered, in a particular social context, rather than adopting a generalised image of the market or marketplace. This was the kind of approach that Jenner and Wallis would later recommend. They see it as a way of exploring the social and economic networks behind healing activities, and as a way of bridging what they call 'the excessively sharp distinctions drawn in the historiography between the English medical marketplace and European medical pluralism'.[25] Unfortunately, Jenner and Wallis say virtually nothing about the latter and, rather confusingly, of the two examples they provide of it (Katherine Park and Gianna Pomata), neither actually used pluralism as a model.[26]

Perhaps this is the dilemma: despite the significant points the two models have in common, they will continue to remain distinct – favouring an economic interpretation of the interaction between patient and practitioner, the other a cultural one. There is certainly a case to be made that the two approaches can learn from one another, the marketplace becoming more 'cul-

25   Jenner/Wallis (2007), pp. 16–17.
26   Park (1985); Pomata (1998).

tural', and the pluralism model giving more consideration to the 'economic'. That said, I would not wish to go so far as one recent economically-minded critic, who has called medical pluralism an 'illusion'. Gil-Soo Han has noted that, like biomedicine, traditional and non-orthodox medicines reflect the dominant capitalist mode of production.[27] They in fact resemble biomedicine, despite occasional lingering pre-capitalist modes of production. Like biomedicine, they exhibit features of professionalisation: their practice is fee-for-service, knowledge and skills based, commodified (relying on medication), and institutionalised. But Han is too dismissive of the pluralism exhibited by past societies.[28] His critique may pose difficulties for the use of the pluralism model in the present, though even this is debatable; but it does not invalidate its applicability for early modern Italy.

Bibliography

Bamji, Alexandra: Religion and Disease in Venice, c. 1620–1700. Diss. University of Cambridge 2007.

Cook, Harold: The Decline of the Old Medical Regime in Stuart London. Ithaca, NY 1986.

Deacon, Harriet: The Cape Doctor and the Broader Medical Market, 1800–1850. In: Deacon, Harriet; Phillips, Howard; Van Heyningen, Elizabeth (eds.): The Cape Doctor in the Nineteenth Century. Amsterdam 2004, pp. 45–84.

Gentilcore, David: Healers and Healing in Early Modern Italy. Manchester 1998.

Gentilcore, David: Ritualized Illness and Music Therapy. Views of Tarantism in the Kingdom of Naples. In: Horden, Peregrine (ed.): Music as Medicine: the History of Music Therapy since Antiquity. London 2000, pp. 255–272.

Gentilcore, David: Fu Guarito, e Perfettamente, Dalla musica: Epifanio Ferdinando e il Tarantismo Pugliese. In Marti, Mario; Urgesi, Domenico (eds.): Epifanio Ferdinando, Medico e Storico del Seicento. Nardò 2001, pp. 134–148.

Gentilcore, David: Charlatans, the Regulated Marketplace and the Treatment of Venereal Disease in Italy. In: Siena, Kevin (ed.): Sins of the Flesh. Responding to Sexual Disease in Early Modern Europe. Toronto 2005, pp. 57–80.

Gentilcore, David: Medical Charlatanism in Early Modern Italy. Oxford 2006.

Goubert, Jean-Pierre: Twenty Years On. Problems of Historical Methodology in the History of Health. In: Porter, Roy; Wear, Andrew (eds.): Problems and Methods in the History of Medicine. London 1987, pp. 40–56.

Han, Gil-Soo: The Myth of Medical Pluralism. A Critical Realist Perspective. In: Sociological Research Online 6 (2002), no. 4, available at: http://www.socresonline.org.uk/6/4/han.html (accessed 5 December 2012).

27 Han (2002), paragraph 6.11.
28 Han dismisses the presence of 'avocational' healers described by anthropologists like Charles Leslie. Leslie (1980), pp. 192–193. Healers who are not full-time professionals, possessing other forms of status and income, may once haved existed in isolated tribal societies, Han says; but globalisation has meant that 'being avocational medical practitioners becomes nearly impossible under the present modes of political economy'. Han (2002), paragraph 6.3.

Henry, John: Doctors and Healers. Popular Culture and the Medical Profession. In: Pumfrey, Stephen; Rossi, Paolo L.; Slawinski, Maurice (eds.): Science, Culture and Popular Belief in Renaissance Europe. Manchester 1991, pp. 191–221.

Jenner, Mark; Wallis, Patrick (eds.): Medicine and the Market in England and its Colonies, c.1450–c.1850. Basingstoke 2007.

Kleinman, Arthur: Concepts and a Model for the Comparison of Medical Systems as Cultural Systems. In: Social Science and Medicine 12 (1978), pp. 85–93.

Kleinman, Arthur: Patients and Healers in the Context of Culture. An Exploration of the Borderland between Anthropology, Medicine, and Pyschiatry. Berkeley 1980.

Leslie, Charles: Medical Pluralism in World Perspectives. In: Social Science and Medicine 14 B (1980), pp. 191–195.

López Terrada, María Luz: Medical Pluralism in the Iberian Kingdoms. The Control of Extra-Academic Practitioners in Valencia. In: Medical History Supplement 29 (2007), pp. 7–25.

Nutton, Vivian: Healers in the Medical Market Place. Towards a Social History of Graeco-Roman Medicine. In: Wear, Andrew (ed.): Medicine in Society. Cambridge 1992, pp. 15–58.

Papadopoulos, Christos: The Greek World and Medical Tradition. Healers and Healing on the Eve of the Greek Revival (1700–1821). Diss. University College London 2008.

Park, Katherine: Doctors and Medicine in Early Modern Florence. Princeton 1985.

Pomata, Gianna: Contracting a Cure. Patients, Healers and the Law in Early Modern Bologna. Baltimore 1998.

Rubel, Arthur; O'Nell, Carl; Collado-Ardón, Rolando: Susto, a Folk Illness. Berkeley 1984.

Whitaker, Elizabeth: The Idea of Health. History, Medical pluralism, and the Management of the Body in Emilia-Romagna, Italy. In: Medical Anthropology Quarterly N.S. 17 (2003), no. 3, pp. 348–375.

Medical Pluralism in Early Modern France

Matthew Ramsey

The term 'medical pluralism' is widely used to refer to the coexistence of different types of medical practitioners and of divergent and sometimes incompatible medical practices and beliefs, which may or may not be limited to certain types of practitioners. Pluralism often implies as well a pattern in which patients have recourse to different practitioners and treatments, and in a broader and more complex sense to what Waltraud Ernst has called 'the plural or multi-dimensional qualities inherent in medical practices and experiences, as they draw on and are open to different approaches'.[1]

Medical pluralisms: Present and Past

The term first gained currency in the late 1970s, in the work of anthropologists.[2] The key figure was Charles Leslie, a specialist on Asian medicine, who engaged his colleagues in discussions of the concept at conferences and in edited volumes. He writes that 'medical systems are pluralistic structures of different kinds of practitioners and institutional norms'.[3] He gives a central place to Robert Redfield's model of the 'great' and 'little' traditions, the first of which was sustained by an educated elite.[4] He applies the label 'great-tradition medicine' to 'three great streams of learned medical practice and theory that originated in the Chinese, South Asian, and Mediterranean civilizations' and were subsequently imported to the Americas. Despite important differences, they had much in common, founded on a humoural theory and linking the human body to the structure and movements of the cosmos.[5] Another key parallel appears in the forms of medical practice: 'All the civilizations with great tradition medical systems developed a range of practitioners from learned professional physicians to individuals who had limited or no formal training and who practised a simplified version of the great tradition medicine'.[6] In addition, 'other healers co-existed with these practitioners, their arts falling into special categories: bone-setters, surgeons, midwives, snake-bite curers, shamans, and so on'.[7]

1   Ernst (2002), quotation p. 9.
2   On the origins and development of the concept and the controversies surrounding it, see Baer (2011).
3   See Leslie: Asian Medical Systems (1976), especially editor's introduction and part IV, 'The culture of plural medical systems'. Quotation p. 9.
4   Redfield (1956).
5   Leslie: Asian Medical Systems (1976), quotation p. 2.
6   Leslie (1974), quotation p. 74.
7   Leslie: Asian Medical Systems (1976), p. 3.

What most scholars refer to as biomedicine, Leslie, borrowing from the medical anthropologist Frederick Dunn, prefers to describe as a fourth tradition, with its own learned practitioners and characteristic beliefs and practices, not regional but worldwide, although it had its historical origins in Europe: 'cosmopolitan medicine'. The label 'scientific' could also be claimed by Ayurvedic medicine in India, Yunani (Graeco-Arabic) and Chinese medicine; 'modern' wrongly implies that the other traditions did not change; 'Western' fails to recognize its global spread and implantation.[8] One characteristic feature of cosmopolitan medicine has been 'the ways in which [it] progressively subordinates other forms of practice'.[9] Only in Asia have the learned traditions survived among educated elites, though typically transformed by borrowings from the institutions and practices of cosmopolitan medicine.[10] Where biomedicine has been more successful in suppressing its rivals, Hans Baer suggests that we speak not of 'pluralistic' but of 'plural' medical systems, which 'may be described as *dominative* in that one medical system, namely biomedicine, enjoys pre-eminent institutional status vis-à-vis other medical systems'. With that proviso, however, he accepts that 'medical pluralism flourishes in all complex or state societies' (as opposed to indigenous tribal societies) and that 'biomedicine's dominance over rival medical systems has never been absolute'.[11] Leslie, however, labels all 'health systems' pluralistic, despite what may in some cases appear to be 'a single, standardized hieratic medical system administered by university-trained physicians'. The United States is no exception. There

> the medical system is composed of physicians, dentists, druggists, clinical psychologists, chiropractors, social workers, health food experts, masseurs, yoga teachers, spirit curers, Chinese herbalists and so on. The health concepts of a Puerto Rican worker in New York City, the curers he consults, and the therapies he receives, differ from those of a Chinese laundryman or a Jewish clerk. These concepts and the practitioners they consult differ in turn from those of middle-class believers in Christian science or in logical positivism.[12]

Over the last three decades, although the concept of medical pluralism has remained in common use, medical anthropologists have challenged the ways in which Leslie and others applied it.[13] The term 'medical system', with its functionalist overtones, implies a degree of consistency and coherence which even biomedicine does not fully possess. The older term 'medical culture' allows for tensions and even contradictions, but the idea that each nation or society has its own distinctive medical culture and subcultures has its own prob-

8   For a defence of the term 'cosmopolitan medicine' and arguments against the alternatives, see Leslie: Asian Medical Systems (1976), pp. 5–8. See also Dunn (1976).
9   Leslie: Asian Medical Systems (1976), p. 6.
10   Leslie: Ambiguities (1976). On pp. 358–359 he describes eight 'types' of medicine in modern India. See also the articles in Ebrahimnejad (2009).
11   Baer (2011), p. 413. Emphasis in original.
12   Leslie: Asian Medical Systems (1976), pp. 9–10.
13   Littlewood (2007). See also Baer (2011), p. 419.

lems.[14] Anthropologists have problematized the concept of culture, in two senses, both as a domain of human activity specifically devoted to the production of meaning, which one can distinguish from other social and political domains; and a set of symbols, rituals, discourses – a culture linked to a particular population, distinguished from others. Critics point, on the one hand, to the omnipresence of meaning in social life, and, on the other, to the extent and frequency of exchanges between human populations, even in non-Western regions that seem very isolated.[15] The second point applies a fortiori to the components (or whatever other term one wishes to apply) that make a pluralistic medical culture pluralistic. Even the notion of syncretism assumes the coherence of preexisting bodies of knowledge and practice that can be combined in new ways. A related concern is the one-to-one correspondence that Leslie sometimes suggests between discrete types of practitioners, the patients who consult them, and shared beliefs and practices, as when he writes in the passage quoted in the previous paragraph about 'the health concepts of a Puerto Rican worker in New York City, the curers he consults, and the therapies he receives'. That worker may be more likely than the stereotypical Chinese laundryman or Jewish clerk to consult a *curandero* in Spanish Harlem who uses holy water and Roman Catholic prayers, but both are also likely to use the services of other practitioners, including those trained in biomedicine, in similar ways.

The sociologists Sarah Cant and Ursula Sharma write that the concept of medical pluralism 'was developed in the context of research on the countries of the South where a biomedical monopoly of health care services has been the exception rather than the rule', and 'different kinds of healing systems exist alongside each other and interact with each other'. They ask to what extent it can be compared to the '"new" medical pluralism in the West', the product of the growing popularity of 'alternative' and 'complementary' medicines, which since the late 1960s have challenged the century-old hegemony of biomedicine. Although the hegemony of biomedicine was never absolute, they see in the late twentieth century the 're-emergence' or 'revival' of an older pattern.[16] An American sociologist, Michael S. Goldstein, similarly writes of the 'persistence and resurgence of medical pluralism' in the United States and also stresses the prominence of CAM (complementary and alternative medicine).[17] The implications and adequacy of labels such as biomedicine, CAM, and various other terms has been the subject of a debate too complex to summarize here, but the prevalence of practices and beliefs that would not appear in a medical school curriculum is not in dispute.[18]

---

14   On the concept of 'medical culture' see Roelcke (1998). On national medical cultures, see Last (1999).
15   Sewell (1999). See also Brightman (1999).
16   Cant/Sharma (1999), pp. 1–4. Emphasis in original.
17   Goldstein (2004). The article is a critique of the sociologist Paul Starr's account of the 'rise of professional sovereignty' (Starr (1982)).
18   On the terminology, see Jütte (2001).

Cant and Sharma propose five categories for sorting out 'non-biomedical modes of healing found in western countries', according to their historical origins: (1) 'those that developed prior to, or contemporaneously with, modern biomedicine', ranging from homoeopathy to 'folk' healing; (2) those, such as chiropractic, which 'originated in the period of medical individualism which characterized health care in America in the late nineteenth and early twentieth century'; (3) those, such as naturopathy, 'derived from the practices of central European health spas that flourished in the nineteenth century'; (4) those, such as acupuncture, 'that re-emerged in the West or were imported by westerners in various versions from Asia'; and (5) those, like Chinese herbal medicine, 'that have entered western countries with immigrant groups' and in some but not all cases have spread outside those populations.[19]

Medical exchanges between the western and non-western worlds moved in both directions.[20] The classifications used by other authors can look quite different, like the 'taxonomy of unconventional healing practices' that David Eisenberg and Ted Kaptchuk present in their analysis of medical pluralism in the United States. One of their categories, 'parochial unconventional medicine', which is associated with particular religions, ethnic groups, and regions, partly overlaps Cant and Sharma's fifth category. It extends beyond recent immigrant groups, however, and they emphasize isolation rather than sharing.[21]

In the United States, a long ethnographic tradition has been devoted to the study of American Indian medicine, African-derived beliefs and practices maintained by slaves and their descendants, and the persistence of distinctive forms of practice and therapies among the Hispanic population, especially in the Southwest.[22] Recent immigrant groups have received similar attention, particularly those from the non-Western world that appear to have resisted cultural assimilation. The *locus classicus* is a book published in 1997 by the writer Anne Fadiman, *The Spirit Catches You and You Fall Down: A Hmong Child, Her American Doctors, and the Collision of Two Cultures.* 'The spirit catches you and you fall down' is a literal translation of the Hmong expression for epilepsy, which makes clear that the Hmong conceptions of this disease and its etiology differ greatly from those of biomedicine. The book deals with the encounters that took place in California in the early 1990s between a community of Laotian refugees and the American system of health care, social services, and justice. The parents of the little girl in question, accused of not following medical advice, wound up losing custody of their child on the grounds of neglect. In the author's view, these incidents showed not only differences in language, values, and behavioural norms between health care personnel, on the one hand, and the family and fellow Hmong on the other, but also the in-

---

19   Cant/Sharma (1999), pp. 5–6.
20   See Bivins (2007).
21   Kaptchuk/Eisenberg: Varieties 1 (2001) and Kaptchuk/Eisenberg: Varieties 2 (2001), quotation p. 200.
22   See Baer (2001), chap. 9: 'Folk Medical Systems in a culturally diverse society'.

commensurability of two systems of medical practices and ideas, indeed two systems of thought. Hence the last phrase in the book's title: 'the collision of two cultures'. Medical pluralism appears as one manifestation of multicultural-ism.[23]

The perception that a better understanding of such differences and a will-ingness to accommodate beliefs and practices specific to an ethnocultural mi-nority when they do not directly conflict with biomedicine has led to a move-ment to promote 'cultural competence' among health providers of various kinds.[24] The main objective is to make providers less likely to blunder when dealing with minority group members, by overcoming their own ethnocen-trism – including their attachment to biomedicine as a cultural system – and more resourceful in finding ways to increase acceptance and compliance. This approach could be called a form of 'integrative medicine', not in the usual sense of a program to incorporate certain unconventional practices and prac-titioners into biomedicine, subject to the standards of 'evidence-based medi-cine', but in the sense of incorporating into biomedicine the patients who share unconventional beliefs about health and illness.[25]

The question whether current complementary and alternative medicines represent a resurgence or simply the persistence of an earlier form of medical pluralism into an era of biomedical dominance assumes that earlier form as a reference point. This approach is neither simple nor unproblematic. One could turn the question around and ask how well a model of pluralism origi-nally applied to non-Western postcolonial societies and then to the West in the twentieth century applies to earlier periods. Biomedicine co-exists outside the West with older traditions, and in the West with various 'alternative' medi-cines, some of them non- Western imports. There are parallels in the nine-teenth century, particularly in the United States, which saw the emergence of coherent alternative medical systems.[26] Some were what I have termed 'counterhegemonic' – explicitly in opposition to the medical profession and medical orthodoxy.[27] For earlier periods, however, we risk anachronism in writing about what Roy Porter, in his analysis of 'quackery' in Georgian Eng-land, called 'fringe medicine before the fringe', before the prominent unortho-dox medical movements of the Victorian age.[28]

All recent scholarship on medicine in early modern Europe recognizes a wide variety of practitioners and practices, but there is no standard vocabulary to describe the larger pattern or the particular variations. Some historians not surprisingly shy away from social science models and typologies that are con-

---

23 Fadiman (1997).
24 See, for example, Lecca et al. (1998), and Purnell/Paulanka (1998).
25 On the integrative medicine movement, see, for example, Scheid/MacPherson (2012). On the evolution of attitudes in the American medical profession: Winnick (2005).
26 See, for example, Baer (2001), chap. 1, 'Nineteenth-Century American Medicine as a Pluralistic System'.
27 Ramsey (1999), p. 289.
28 Porter (1988); Porter (2000), pp. 200–206.

tested by social scientists themselves. Nor is there consistency in the use of 'medical pluralism'. Sometimes it simply denotes variety. Roy Porter, who typically avoids the term, does write of a 'lively medical pluralism' in England in the long eighteenth century, which he attributes to the lack of effective regulation and 'the relative inefficacy of medicine' in the face of rampant disease. Patients tried many different things.[29] The main thrust of his argument, however, emphasizes an open marketplace where remedy vendors of every stripe competed on more or less equal terms and often used very similar therapies. This is not 'pluralism' in the usual sense of the coexistence of distinctive groups or beliefs.[30] In her work on medicine in eighteenth-century Germany and early modern Europe, Mary Lindemann recognizes a profusion of different practitioners and practices – within a widely shared common fund of knowledge. She does not, however, use 'medical pluralism' to frame either her survey of early modern European medicine and society or her monograph on Braunschweig-Wolfenbüttel, though in the latter study she refers in passing to 'a world that nourished quackery and in which medical pluralism flourished'.[31] A central point in both books is that 'few people [...] adhered to one "system" or another, and almost all were medically promiscuous'.[32] (The terms 'promiscuous' and 'promiscuity' appear in works by other historians.[33] Because they suggest indiscriminate behaviour, 'eclectic' might better characterize the choices that patients made in a therapeutic itinerary.) Although factors such as cost and distance imposed real constraints, broadly speaking the socioeconomic status of patients did not dictate the type of practitioner consulted, and the therapies they accepted were not necessarily logically consistent.

Despite the consensus on the multifariousness of practitioners and practices, transposing the modern conceptions of medical pluralism to the early modern period leads to difficulties. One study of 'medical pluralism' in early modern Spain starts with the definition of pluralism as 'the coexistence of medical systems' and states that in this case it 'involves the co-existence of academic medicine – the Galenism taught in universities to physicians, surgeons, and apothecaries through guild-based instruction – and other forms of medical practice [including] alternatives to traditional Galenic therapies'.[34] As the author herself notes, however, some practitioners from outside the corporations often claimed and sometimes actually enjoyed official approval. Their

29 Porter (2000), p. 34.
30 Jenner/Wallis (2007). In their introduction, 'The Medical Marketplace', the editors stress a theme running through the papers collected in the volume: 'it is not always helpful to equate medical pluralism with the medical market' (p. 6).
31 Lindemann (2010); Lindemann (1996), quotation p. 233.
32 Lindemann (2010), p. 305. Cf. Lindemann (1996), p. 241: 'medical promiscuity characterized early modern people'.
33 For example, Burnham (2005), p. 51, quotes Lindemann. Cf. Gentilcore (2006), p. 258: 'people did not differentiate much when it came to the competing claims of different levels of medicine. They were medically promiscuous.'
34 López Terrada (2009), quotations pp. 7–8. As the subtitle indicates, the article focuses on the regulation of medical practice in the various Spanish kingdoms.

therapies, which sometimes resembled those of formally trained practitioners, could better be described as a congeries than a system.

The most systematic and thoughtful discussion of these issues can be found in the work of David Gentilcore on early modern Italy, which is summarized in his contribution to this volume. His first book, on the sacred in the Terra d'Otranto, has a subchapter on medical pluralism; it was followed by a study of medical practitioners and practices in the Kingdom of Naples, which devoted a chapter to medical pluralism.[35] A third work deals with 'charlatanism' and focuses on itinerants who were licensed to sell their drugs; the larger framework of pluralism is assumed but not explicitly developed. One major finding is that the charlatans' therapies were similar to those used by physicians, though as Gentilcore notes, remedies inconsistent with learned medicine 'would not have been licensed'.[36] Pluralism encompasses both practitioners and therapies: 'the range of healers that existed in a time of medical pluralism'; 'in a time of medical pluralism, cures existed outside the strictly medical'.[37] Unlike many colleagues working on related topics, Gentilcore gives extended attention to religious healing. The model that he proposes for medical pluralism is a Venn diagram with three overlapping circles, representing the medical, the ecclesiastical and the popular. The categories include both practitioners and beliefs and practices, and the attitudes of patients as well as practitioners. None is limited to a particular segment of the population, whether physicians for the medical, clergy for the ecclesiastical, or the urban poor and peasants for the popular.[38]

The category of the popular is the least clear and most contested of the three, challenged by, among others, Lindemann for Germany and John Henry for early modern England, who describe a body of knowledge shared by different social groups.[39] In an essay on the concept of popular medicine in early modern Europe, Gentilcore starts by noting the increasing separation of 'learned and popular medicine' in the eighteenth century and asks whether historians of early modern medicine – especially those influenced by the model of the open medical marketplace that Roy Porter describes for Georgian England – are not 'exaggerating its [...] unity'. Such an account 'tends to imply an overly consensual view of what were complex and pluralistic societies, where the pluralism was a source (or symptom?) of deep tensions'. It might be true that 'doctors and patients shared a common language, but this was often because the physicians were bilingual', capable of a kind of cultural competency *avant la lettre*. 'Differences in language reflected real differences in mentality and perception.' It may not be possible to identify a single discrete body of popular medical beliefs and practices, but Gentilcore suggests that it

35 Gentilcore (1992), pp. 129–131; Gentilcore (1998), chap. 1, 'Medical Pluralism in the Kingdom of Naples'.
36 Gentilcore (1998), quotation p. 232.
37 Gentilcore (1998), p. 177; Gentilcore (2006), p. 258.
38 Gentilcore (1998), pp. ix, 3, 203.
39 Lindemann (1996). See also Henry (1991).

would be worth examining the health-related beliefs and practices of various subordinate groups, and, more broadly, 'the nature of cultural exchange between different levels of society'.[40] Gianna Pomata's work on early modern Bologna leads her to similar conclusions about contrasting views of the body, sickness, and therapy held by patients and 'popular healers' on the one hand, and physicians on the other.[41]

The notion of the popular, however defined, is of course only one way to identify differences as well as similarities in early modern medicine. Depending on our angle of vision, we can find different kinds of difference among groups – in institutions, religion, and language and ethnicity, among others, which could affect health-related practices and beliefs. One complication is identifying the geographic unit of analysis, which for studies of modern pluralism is commonly the nation state. Although Lindemann's study of Braunschweig-Wolfenbüttel has 'Germany' in its title, and Gentilcore's work on the Kingdom of Naples the word 'Italy' – perhaps the publisher's decision – each deals with a state before national unification, which occurred in the nineteenth century.[42] Institutional and legal differences with implications for medical practice existed in the Spanish kingdoms, and in England and Wales, Scotland, and Ireland. But political boundaries did not always define the populations or the regional differences we might wish to study.

Early modern France

France in the Old Regime was a kingdom but not a unified nation state like the modern 'Hexagon'. Its boundaries expanded dramatically between the late fifteenth and seventeenth centuries; Lorraine and Corsica were added in the eighteenth century. Although the Crown sought to impose its authority and establish greater administrative uniformity throughout its territories, the new provinces retained institutions, laws, languages, and culture. Local and regional identities remained stronger than any sense of being 'French'.[43] It has been estimated that in 1789 half the population did not speak French. They were concentrated in the peripheral provinces, where regional languages and dialects unrelated or not closely related to French, predominated – Breton (a Celtic language), Basque (not even an Indo-European language), Alsatian (a Low Alemannic German dialect), and the West Flemish dialect of Dutch, among others. The French revolutionaries saw linguistic diversity as a major

---

40 Gentilcore (2004), quotations pp. 159, 162.
41 Pomata (1998), p. 135 and passim.
42 Lindemann (1996) suggests that Braunschweig-Wolfenbüttel was similar to 'most other small to medium-sized secular German states' (p. 19).
43 An extended exploration of how France became a unified kingdom can be found in Braudel (1988–1990). For a brief summary, see Beik (2009), subchapter 'The Creation of France', pp. 1–4. Jones (1994).

obstacle to the development of a national identity.[44] In religion, France was sharply divided between Roman Catholics and Protestants, mainly Calvinists; the Lutherans in the northeast enjoyed a special status though not always full de facto toleration. Following the bitter wars of religion that had begun in 1562, the Edict of Nantes, issued by Henri IV in 1598, granted significant rights to Protestants without ending the special status of the Catholic Church. The revocation of the edict by Louis XIV in 1685 led to a massive emigration of Protestants and provoked an insurrection in the Cévennes mountains in south-central France (1702–1710).[45]

These cultural differences affected health-related practices and beliefs, as well as the relations of patients with practitioners, without constituting separate medical 'systems'.[46] It is hard to find close analogies to Eisenberg and Kaptchuk's 'parochial unconventional medicine'. One can of course point to examples of small marginalized communities strongly marked as 'other' by language, religion, and customs – the Jews, who were expelled and then recalled several times in the Middle Age and began returning in small numbers in the seventeenth century, or the Romani people, who entered France starting in the early fifteenth century. Jews played a disproportionate role as learned physicians in Christian and Muslim countries, despite some restrictions in the former. Their communities also preserved other practices quite distinct from classical medicine, including some linked to religious obligations, and other elements like charms that we would label magical.[47] Romani medicine is based on a particular cosmology in which disease is attributed to *marimé*, that which is morally or physically impure, or to Mamioro, a spirit attracted by dirty houses.[48] But in the main, we are dealing with major similarities as well as differences, leaving the significance of both open to interpretation. Moreover, despite some differences, medical institutions across the kingdom shared a corporatist form of organization.[49] France had no royal or state regulatory body in the health field comparable to the *protomedicatos* of Italy, Spain and the Spanish Empire.[50]

Discussions of both medical practitioners and practices in Old Regime France have been heavily influenced by the massive synthetic work published in 1997 by Laurence Brockliss and Colin Jones, *'The Medical World of Early Modern France'*.[51] It is regularly referenced in discussions of medical pluralism, extending beyond the history of France and the world of Anglo-American historiography, although the authors themselves use the term itself only once, to describe the breakdown of doctrinal consensus among the medical elite

---

44   See Bell (2001), chap. 6, 'National Language and the Revolutionary Crucible'.
45   Carbonnier-Burkard/Cabanel (1998).
46   See, for example, Goubert (1974).
47   Shatzmiller (1994); Zimmels (1997).
48   Bowness (1970).
49   Ramsey (1988), chap. l; Brockliss/Jones (1997), chap. 3.
50   On the *protomedicato*, see, for example, Gentilcore (1999) and Lanning/TePaske (1985).
51   Brockliss/Jones (1997).

over the course of the eighteenth century.[52] Parts of what follows will unavoidably have a polemical tone, because despite masterly treatments of many other topics, ranging from medical education to the history of disease, the work is in some ways problematic on the questions at issue here.

Confronted with the blur and confusion of practitioners, some officially authorized in various ways and others not, the authors propose what they call 'a relatively new set of terms and concepts to structure our findings', starting with 'medical world [...] a term by which we designate the whole set of practitioners of health services, trained and untrained, educated and non-educated, male and female, working in France between the sixteenth century and the French Revolution'. Within that world they locate a

> central institutional core of medical orthodoxy, [around which] there was [...] a penumbra of practitioners socially or institutionally associated to a greater or lesser extent with the central core and dominated more or less loosely by the ideas of the orthodox medical community.[53]

I would note in passing, since Brockliss and Jones cite my own work as a foil to their interpretation, that my discussion of the social world of medical practice in the Old Regime devotes a subchapter to the 'great penumbra' of practitioners outside the medical corporations who enjoyed some degree of legal recognition.[54] To see my own terminology offered as part of what is presented as a corrective is one of the most perplexing historiographical moves I have encountered. There are some differences: the Brockliss-Jones penumbra embraces absolutely everyone outside the core, and the social and institutional links to the core become increasingly tenuous. Their account of medical practice is urban and to a large degree Paris-centric, and much of France remains in the shadows. For many inhabitants of France, the core and especially the capital were in a sense the periphery.

In the eighteenth century, the authors describe the emergence of 'new forms of entrepreneurialism' and 'the development of a medical marketplace in the capital' for the sale of proprietary remedies not very different from Porter's account of the market in eighteenth-century England. This new marketplace included 'practitioners on the margins of the orthodox medical community', though we are never told what percentage of physicians, surgeons, and apothecaries participated. The entrepreneurial free-for-all tended to undermine the authority of the medical corporations. As Porter argues in the English case, market competition blurred the distinctions among different types of practitioners.[55] In an article published a year before the book, Jones shows how a new periodical press helped extend the reach of the market into the

---

52 See, for example, Perdiguero (1994); Zarzoso (2001); Brockliss/Jones (1997), p. 27.
53 Brockliss/Jones (1997), pp. 8, 237.
54 Ramsey (1988), pp. 31–38. Porter (1986), p. 16, used the term 'penumbra' in a similar sense – 'a perennial penumbra of respected and tolerated irregulars' – even earlier but did not develop the concept.
55 Brockliss/Jones (1997), 'Medical Entrepreneurialism in the Enlightenment'.

provinces.[56] The concept of a medical marketplace in France is hardly new.[57] The very prominent place that Brockliss and Jones assign to remedy vending in this context as opposed to all other forms of health-related practices is distinctive, however.

Much of the Brockliss-Jones argument concerns something else – the ideas that dominate what they see as a 'unitary world' or 'unitary medical universe'. 'To a very considerable extent,' they write, 'especially in the sixteenth and seventeenth centuries, trained and untrained practitioners participated in a shared medical discourse.'[58] Like their model of medical practice, this view has won broad acceptance.[59] Gentilcore has been one of the few prominent dissenters.[60] In the realm of practices and beliefs, Brockliss and Jones see a widely shared understanding of the body, health, and disease characterized by Galenic principles. Though elsewhere they seek to eschew the labels popular and elite, they write of a 'popular Galenism' derived from 'the learned culture of the elite'. They write that

> in examining the admittedly very partial, incomplete, and skewed records that we have of popular medicine at the furthest extreme from the core of the orthodox medical community, we frequently meet ideas and beliefs which have started off as conventional medical doctrines and which have subsequently become lodged in systems of general belief [...].

They allow that medical ideas common among the lower classes had sources other than Galenism, 'notably oral tradition, collective memory and folkloric precedent', and characterize certain religious healing practices as 'folkloric in the extreme'. They concede that 'we can be pretty sure that the further we are away from the literate medical core', the more prevalent were other ideas about health and healing. Nevertheless, they characterize these beliefs, quoting Keith Thomas, as 'the debris of many different systems of thought'; 'much popular medicine was out-of-date or misunderstood élite medicine'. They renounce any

> attempt to inventorize, let alone genealogize or describe, the extraordinary range of beliefs about healing held by some people some of the time in early modern France (indeed, we have a healthy scepticism about the viability of such a task on the basis of the sources available).[61]

No one, to my knowledge, has identified a completely autonomous and distinctive corpus of practices and beliefs that could be labelled popular medicine. The ways in which the armamentarium of physicians overlapped with that of many untrained practitioners and remedy vendors is well known. But even apart from the many practices that do not fit the Galenic model, several caveats are in order. Different practitioners who employ the same treatment

---

56 Jones (1996).
57 See, for example, Ramsey (1988).
58 Brockliss/Jones (1997), pp. 17, 283.
59 See, for example, Stein (2009), p. 15, and Herzlich (2001), pp. 28–29.
60 Gentilcore (2004), pp. 158, 162.
61 Brockliss/Jones (1997), pp. 17–18, 79, 273–275. Quotation from Thomas (1971), p. 185.

may have different ways of diagnosing disease and employing the therapy. Peasants in eighteenth-century Brittany might purge themselves once a year and during certain illnesses; but one physician who prescribed purgatives during an epidemic of dysentery and met with resistance complained that he could not make these ignorant rustics understand that the quality of the evacuations mattered as much as the quantity.[62] The meanings of what is seemingly the same therapy can change over time, as the context changes. In their search for learned antecedents, Brockliss and Jones sometimes come perilously close to anachronism. Take the case of a parish priest in the Alps in the nineteenth century who reportedly treated a patient with an intestinal worm by suspending him upside down over a bowl of warm milk and seizing the worm when it emerged to drink the milk. Jones points to a print taken from a late fifteenth-century vernacular surgical text which he found reproduced in an old medical history textbook. It shows the same procedure, proving its 'impeccable ancestry in learned culture'. Yet many of the priest's contemporaries not surprisingly regarded the treatment as a form of popular medicine, a term that was coming into increasing use among physicians and other writers on medical subjects.[63]

Just as Brockliss and Jones cannot avoid invoking practices that 'had their roots in popular traditions' as opposed to Galenic medicine, they cannot avoid noticing differences that might separate some practitioners from many of their potential patients. They quote a rural physician who complained that the people would always turn to a local healer rather than a physician.

> The author of these lines was quite correct in registering the continued presence of large numbers of local healers, whose hold over the rural populations would last well into the nineteenth century. Yet when he sententiously concluded 'we naturally like what resembles us, and we are loth to listen to an individual we don't understand', he was missing the point. For what was striking about the place of medicine in the rural world in the eighteenth century was less the continued presence of local healers and wise women than the penetration of the rural milieu by large numbers of itinerant practitioners [many of them primarily remedy vendors] stressing difference from – rather than similarity to – local populations.[64]

The key point is that we need to be attuned to differences as well as similarities. They need not be radical. Sometimes small variations that can be significant cultural markers, like local idioms in a shared language. A given practice can be open to divergent interpretations, reflecting differences in perspective but also contests for authority and control. This question is best approached by looking at particular encounters, not between medical systems but between people – practitioners and patients, practitioners and other practitioners.

---

62 Jean-Guillaume Chifoliau, 'Préjugés opposées aux sages précautions du gouvernement, aux efforts des ministres de la santé, et à la voix de la nature', Saint-Malo, 22 March 1780, Archives of the Société Royale de Médecine (at the Académie Nationale de Médecine, Paris, SRM 115B-204).

63 Brockliss/Jones (1997), pp. 18, 275, and Jones (1990). The textbook is Guthrie (1946). Plate 26 reproduces an illustration from Brunschwig (1497). Cf. Ramsey (1988), p. 228.

64 Brockliss/Jones (1997), pp. 132, 645–646.

A case study

As an illustration, I would like to revisit a *cause célèbre* from sixteenth-century Anjou involving a woman healer, which over time has been invoked to support a variety of arguments.[65] The case was an early confirmation of the broad principle of professional monopoly in medicine; one central issue in the trials was whether the corporate authority of the medical faculty of Angers extended outside its urban seat, or whether French jurisprudence would recognize a special category of rural medical practice among a population that was far removed from physicians and in any case (it was said) rarely needed elaborate therapies to treat their relatively simple diseases.[66] In his celebrated treatise on witchcraft and demonology, the jurist Jean Bodin characterizes the practitioner, whom he mistakenly identifies as an old Italian woman, as a witch-healer and compares her to the *saludadors* of Spain.[67] Starting in the seventeenth century and continuing well into the nineteenth, the case was also cited, quite mistakenly, as a precedent in support of a policy barring women from the practice of medicine.[68] Most recently, in the fullest account of the case to date, which invokes the concept of 'medical pluralism', Susan Broomhall has provided a feminist reading.[69]

Brockliss and Jones cite the case as one of the best documented examples of 'popular Galenism' in early modern France. Their argument is not without some equivocation; they concede that in this case 'there might be differences over diagnosis and therapeutics', and that the links between 'learned medicine and the wider society' not only fostered the spread of the concepts of learned medicine but also 'helped to keep orthodox practitioners in touch with other systems of belief'. Indeed, 'it was still possible for trained physicians to learn from those outside the orthodox medical community, and to accept and adapt ideas coming from outside the charmed circle of Galenic medicine'. Nevertheless, the authors create a portrait of an unauthorized practitioner who had more in common than not with the physicians who brought her to court. Despite the battles over the right to practice, her relationship with the physicians was 'surprisingly mimetic'; such healers 'appear to have shared much of the same world of medical discourse as their learned confrères'. That there was some degree of overlap is undeniable, but the evidence in this case comes from legal arguments presented in court, and the authors' interpretation de-

65   A summary of the case can be found in Villiers (1904), pp. 367–369.
66   This point was picked up by the jurist René Choppin (1608), author of the great customal of Anjou; he cited the Lescallier case in his treatise on the rights of country-dwellers, pp. 164–165.
67   Bodin (1587), fol. 142v.
68   See, for example, Garnier (1937), p. 43.
69   Broomhall (2004), chap. 4, 'Female healing before the law'; quotation p. 5. Her thorough account is based on Bibliothèque nationale de France (henceforth BNF) ms. Baluze 222, 'Playdr de M. Matras et Marion sur une femme qui exercoit la Medecine en lannee 1573', and BNF ms. Français 2137, 'Arrest notable qui defend a une femme d'Anjou d'exercer la medecine, 18 avril 1578'.

pends in part on taking at face value the statements made by one side and dismissing or ignoring those made by their adversaries.[70]

Jeanne Lescallier was a peasant woman who practised medicine in the parish of Denée on the Loire, about 15 kilometres from Angers. Her patients included peasants, artisans, and bourgeois from the provincial capital. She enjoyed an enviable reputation as a bonesetter, generally considered a masculine calling because of the great physical strength it required. She apparently worked for two decades unmolested in the 1550s and 1560s, until an autopsy performed on one of her patients, a barrister of Angers, led to an accusation of poisoning.

The medical faculty denounced her to the authorities of the *sénéchaussée* of Anjou, not for poisoning but for unauthorized medical practice. She was convicted in 1571 and forbidden to practice medicine or surgery, under threat of fines and summary imprisonment. She appealed, and her case eventually reached the *parlement* of Paris, with a large number of inhabitants of her parish and three neighbouring parishes joining her as co-appellants. In April 1573, the council of the *parlement* reached a decision unfavourable to Jeanne, which was confirmed five years later by a royal decree. During all this time, Jeanne appears to have continued to practice, despite the formal prohibitions.[71]

In the episode leading to the intervention of the Angers faculty, the barrister's widow testified that she had called in Jeanne to treat her ailing husband, and that the healer had accepted on condition that she be given free rein and that physicians be excluded from treating the patient. Lescallier made potions of 'strange substances'. For one of these she required a live crow, which she tore apart, placing one half on the patient's head. (Variations on this old procedure long survived in the French countryside, usually in the form of a pigeon placed on the head of a meningitis patient to draw off the poisons.)[72] The other half of the crow she boiled down to a residue, which she worked with a mortar. To this substance she added mistletoe found on oak and a substance she identified as human brain. The whole concoction, after distillation in an alembic, was to be taken internally for nine consecutive days – and would have been, except that the patient died after only two or three. An autopsy revealed 'excoriations' on the viscera, and, according to the examiners, other signs of poisoning.

It was Jeanne's misfortune to have unsuccessfully treated a prominent bourgeois of Angers; the fatal outcome triggered a confrontation with the faculty, which challenged her practice on more general grounds than the one

---

70   Brockliss/Jones (1997), pp. 275–277; the case is also mentioned on pp. 296 and 337. The authors cite BNF ms. Français 18767, fols. 302–309, hearing and judgement of the *parlement* of Paris, 18 April 1578.

71   The account that follows is based on BNF ms. Français 21737, Delamare collection on medicine and surgery, fols. 302r–309r, and ms. français 24055, 'Pièces et arrêts divers de la fin du XVIe', fols 213r-275v. The two manuscripts give the arguments and sentence, in slightly different form, for the appellate trial in 1573. See also LeVest (1612), no. CLVII, 9 April 1573.

72   Bouteiller (1966), p. 256.

case of possible involuntary homicide. Lescallier came under attack on three points: that she was not regularly authorized to practice medicine; that medicine was in any case *officium virile*, not to be taken up by any woman; and that her work itself should be condemned as witchcraft and imposture. On the second question, it should be added, the faculty's argument was inconsistent. Its syndic maintained at one point that the physicians in no way wished to exclude women, 'who have the mind for any science', provided that they were properly trained. This view seems close to that of some humanists in the middle third of the sixteenth century who tried to promote women's education.

Jeanne's defence relied on presenting her activities as similar to the long accepted charitable work of pious elite women who served the sick poor. On the question of her lack of credentials, her advocate, René Bautru, sieur des Matras, a prominent barrister and future mayor of Angers, admitted that she was not formally trained but submitted that not 'title and profession' but good results make a physician. On the second point, he made the dubious claim that women had always been tolerated and even admitted to regular practice and honoured, in Paris and elsewhere. On the question of witchcraft, finally, Jeanne categorically denied the allegation. She had not used imprecations or spells. She could not be a witch, or she would have offended the very neighbours who had rallied to her support. As for rumours of other occult practices, such as cartomancy, they were mere calumnies.

Rather than rely on witchcraft, her defence maintained, Jeanne used oils, waters and herbs and administered all her remedies with prayers, in the name of the Trinity. If God had given her the 'grace' to heal, others should not envy her. God had endowed the simplest among the people with a healing power, recognized long ago even by the pagan emperors. As for the particular remedies she administered to the unfortunate barrister, she had used human skull rather than brain, a remedy that could be found at any apothecary's; crow as a medicine was described in the ancient authors; and mistletoe could also be found in the medical books. One part of her defence claimed that she had learned the art of healing from a great lady, who provided the sort of charitable care sanctioned by the physicians, and had even closely observed physicians at work when she was a young woman in Gascony and the province of Ferrara. Jeanne treated only patients who did not have access to physicians or whom the physicians had abandoned, and she accepted no payment for her services.

The claims concerning Jeanne's therapies do have some basis in the medical literature. A century later, Nicolas Lémery's standard work on pharmacy (1698), reprinted well into the eighteenth century, still mentioned the woody part of mistletoe as a medicine to strengthen the brain and to treat epilepsy, paralysis, apoplexy, lethargy, convulsions, and worms – though he warned that the berries were a violent purgative and possible poison, which inflamed the viscera. Similarly, skull, like many body parts and secretions, figured prominently in the old pharmacopoeia. Lémery mentions skull, preferably from a young man of good temperament who had died a violent death, powdered and taken internally.[73] Indications included epilepsy, apoplexy, and other brain diseases, on the principle of similitude; it was also said to stop diarrhea and promote perspiration. The dispensaries also mention crow, taken internally – entire little ones, or the brains of large ones; it was good against epilepsy and gout. Crow dung was recommended for cough and toothache in children. The perceived value of crow was based in part on the observation that the crow eats the brains of carrion first; hence remedies prepared from it are good for brain disorders.

The physicians, through their advocate Simon Marion, a barrister of the *parlement* of Paris, cited complaints of *maleficium*, noted that Lescallier was commonly known as Jeanne *la devineresse* (diviner-healer) and asserted that she had been prohibited several times from using superstitious practices and evil spells, an allegation that remained undocumented.[74] Their central contention, however, was that they had found no evidence of successful cures, and that if Jeanne did somehow cure her patients, it could not be through natural means.

Either Jeanne could not lay claim to the good results that supposedly trumped university training and official authorization, or else these results had a profoundly illegitimate basis. Leaving jurisprudence aside, the plaintiffs developed an elaborate analysis of Jeanne's reputed healing powers, following a model that appears in other trials of other unauthorized practitioners in the late sixteenth and early seventeenth centuries. If, indeed, she cured, it could be in only one of five ways: (1) through learned medical knowledge, humanly acquired; (2) through medical knowledge divinely infused, analogous to the wisdom of Solomon, or the knowledge of military strategy that another Jeanne, Joan of Arc, had received from on high; (3) through usage and experience, called empiricism by the Greeks; (4) by special grace from God, in the form of a miracle, like the work of the healing saints, or the power of the divinely anointed kings of France to cure scrofula with their touch; or (5) by communication with evil spirits, called *sortilège*, or witchcraft. The faculty's brief seems to have followed Aquinas and others in suggesting that one cannot cure through words or other extraordinary remedies without the help of demons.

Regarding the first possibility, learned medical knowledge, the faculty cited Jeanne's own confession that she had never studied medicine. Jeanne's general ignorance of medical art and theory had emerged in a sort of oral examination conducted by the faculty; when she was asked to give a natural explanation of remedies, she sounded like 'a blind person talking about colours'. She could not therefore have such knowledge directly imparted by God – a claim that Jeanne in any case had never made. On the question of experience, the physicians were less concerned to demonstrate that Jeanne lacked practical knowledge, which she obviously possessed, than to argue that it was grossly

---

73   Lémery (1716), pp. 173, 175, 574.
74   In addition to the compilations mentioned earlier, the arguments for the faculty can be found in Simon Marion, 'Plaidoyer de Messire Simon Marion contre Jehanne la Devineresse', Bibliothèque Municipale d'Orléans, ms. 698, no. 15. See Turgeon (1923).

insufficient. Mere empirics blindly prescribed the same drugs for similar symptoms and lacked the grasp of theory and clinical acumen needed to treat individual cases. Marion then dismissed Jeanne's claims of miraculous healing powers as arrogant, an insult both to the saints and to the glorious kings of France, whose healing gift was a well-attested miracle. Jeanne, unlike true miraculous healers, used drugs and accepted money. 'Miracle' is perhaps a strong word for Jeanne's notion of healing through a special gift – she did not liken herself to a saint any more than to Joan of Arc – but her notion of special divine 'grace' lent itself to this misreading.

Thus, the other four possibilities having been eliminated, it followed that Jeanne used witchcraft to cure, or did not cure at all. Her treatments in any case were not in keeping with health, but smacked of corruption; her remedies were 'superstitious' and 'full of witchcraft and spells'. Human brain, live crow, and mistletoe were all known for their association with evil spirits; mistletoe was used by the Druids; the injunction to take a remedy nine times betokened a superstitious mind. And here gender does figure significantly: women are more susceptible to witchcraft than men; Jeanne's sex increased the probability that she was guilty of the offense. These points came as a kind of climax to the faculty's argument. The charge of witchcraft was seemingly more damning than that of unauthorized medical practice, though Jeanne was never formally accused of that crime.

It is true that mistletoe was traditionally associated with the Druids. Pliny recommended it for purging and then fattening cattle, but treated as a Gaulish superstition its reputation as an antidote.[75] In early modern Europe it was considered to have contraceptive properties. The symbolic significance of the crow is more complex. In a widespread dualistic cosmology, the world was divided between God's and the devil's creations: sun and moon; sheep and goat; dove or pigeon and crow. The bird split in two and applied to the head was normally a pigeon, a good substance used to draw off an evil one; but demonic plants and animals also had their uses as remedies, just as poisons did.[76]

The possible meanings of several of Jeanne's practices are thus ambiguous; no clear line can be drawn between popular and official medicine, or medicine and the occult arts. Some of the same remedies might have been prescribed by a local surgeon for brain fever or nervous disorders. On the other hand, taking the medicine for nine days, with its suggestions of a novena and numerological magic, did smack if not of witchcraft then at least of superstition, in the eyes of the medical elite. As for the brain-eating crow, the treatise on popular medical errors by Laurent Joubert, dean of the medical faculty of Montpellier, first published in 1578 – the end of the decade in which Jeanne's trials occurred – sharply condemned the use of remedies based on a resemblance or analogy between the remedy and the medical condition, such

75   Pliny (1938–1963), vol. 5, book 16, chaps. 93–95.
76   Bouteiller (1966), p. 254.

as the use of a rose of Jericho to aid in childbirth.[77] Moreover, the testimony of witnesses convincingly showed that Jeanne practiced divination to predict the future and find lost objects, and that she claimed a divine healing gift. In a sense the physicians may have been right: Jeanne was a witch. Not that she cast spells, much less attended witches' sabbaths or had intercourse with the devil, as described in learned writings on witchcraft; but she had all the characteristics of a local cunning woman or white witch.

What are we to make of this preoccupation with witchcraft? In a sense it was irrelevant to the case before the courts, which concerned unauthorized medical practice. The charges brought by the faculty and the royal *procureur* did not include criminal witchcraft, and although Jeanne's ordeal coincided with a wave of witchcraft trials in other parts of France and a spate of writings urging intensified repression of witches, from Jean Bodin, Nicolas Rémy, and others, there is no evidence that she herself was ever prosecuted for this offense. It is possible, however, that she might have been treated differently had her case come before the courts a decade later, during the great wave of witchcraft prosecutions that began in the 1580s.[78]

By way of contrast, consider the case of Simon Achard, a 'physician empiric', who appeared before the *présidial* court at Marsillac-en-Poitou during that later period, in 1596, charged with 'magic and necromancy'. Achard said that he had cured and lifted a spell on a certain Lamoyeux and his wife with the help of masses, the Holy Ghost, and the sacrament of marriage, which he had performed for his patients, as well as the laying on of hands by a priest. Under pressure from the court, he admitted that he used a familiar, whom he paid for the cures that he worked. At the same time he claimed, like Jeanne, to have a 'gift of grace'; unlike her, he had obtained it not from God but indirectly from masters of magic in Toledo, Spain, to whom he sent a contribution each year. His main activity, he claimed, was identifying witches, thieves, and other malefactors. He insisted that a woman patient had been bewitched by the sprinkling of certain powders on her buttocks, and that he had rightfully accused her tormentor. Achard was condemned to die, despite his offer to renounce witchcraft and repent, and the sentence was upheld on appeal. Although Achard was described as an empiric, the court never examined his right to heal in itself; his offenses were subsumed under the rubric of necromancy or witchcraft.[79]

---

77 Joubert (1578), and Joubert (1579).
78 See Muchembled (1987).
79 Lancre (1622), pp. 774–785 (among the 'arrests divers et notables contre les sorciers'). Another version of the same case appears in Porcheron (1923), pp. 41–42, attributed to de Lancre's work, although it contains details not included in the copy I consulted. Achard admits religious healing, but he adds that he has treated jaundice using the *loriot*, or golden oriole (by the doctrine of *similia similibus*, a yellow bird might cure a disease that produced yellow symptoms). The court argued that if Achard had cured his patients, it could only have been through necromancy; if the oriole were truly effective, princes and great lords would have sought it out, instead of resorting to Achard as the healer had

The Lescallier and Achard cases represent two ends of a spectrum comprising the work of the cunning people known in French as *devins-guérisseurs*. Jeanne practiced a great deal of medicine, some of it not far removed from what a country surgeon might have prescribed; indeed, she was able to present testimonials on her behalf from several barber-surgeons, though none from physicians. She also practiced a little divination; despite the faculty allusions to *maleficium* and previous trouble with the courts, there is no clear evidence of casting spells or even of lifting them. If one credits the reported public testimony of Achard, even allowing for the pressure placed on him to meet the expectations of his accusers, it would seem that he worked primarily as a counter-witch and may occasionally have administered remedies. Though never directly accused of casting spells, Achard seems far more closely associated than Jeanne with the diabolical arts.

And yet there is also a sense in which Achard, who was executed for witchcraft, and Jeanne, who was never even tried for it, occupy the same ground. In Jeanne's trials, it was crucial to the faculty's case to delegitimize her work by showing that it was not only unauthorized but inherently demonic. Stuart Clark has called attention to the central importance of demonology for early modern intellectuals – not just theologians and magistrates, but also political theorists, students of natural history, and many others, including medical men.[80] For the physicians, still several generations removed from the 'retreat of Satan' described by Robert Mandrou in his classic study of witchcraft in seventeenth-century France, commerce with the devil was at least an intellectual possibility.[81] It recurs as a theme in contemporary writings on popular medical errors and superstitions. It is difficult to know exactly how much weight to assign to this particular argument in a rhetorical exercise designed to disparage one's opponent by any means possible. But it is almost surely the case that the physicians found her activities (which, as Jeanne argued, posed no direct threat to their livelihood) profoundly disturbing.

The confrontation brings into relief a conflict between certain learned and popular views of magical healing. In recent years, a broad distinction between popular and elite culture of the sort presented in synthetic studies by Peter Burke and Robert Muchembled has increasingly fallen out of favor.[82] The overlapping medical practices shared by Jeanne and the learned medical tradition are one illustration of why this should be the case. The much-vexed question of the relationship between learned demonology and popular witchcraft beliefs is another.[83] For Jeanne and at least some of her patients, her mi-

---

claimed. In this version, as in the first, the court does not directly question the defendant's right to heal.

80   Clark (1997).
81   Mandrou (1968).
82   Burke (1978); Muchembled (1985).
83   Something of the difficulty of this problem is suggested by two essays in Briggs (1989). First, a more general essay embraces the prevalent view that 'diabolism was never more than a secondary, even an imposed element in peasant belief' ('Witchcraft and the Community in France and French-speaking Europe', p. 15), but a second, monographic essay

raculous healing powers were both real and clearly beneficent; they could neither be explained through the ordinary laws of nature nor attributed to the devil; 'divine grace' was her somewhat inadequate attempt to account for the phenomenon. She could not be a witch, for witches by definition harmed their neighbors.

The physicians' discourse, in common with most French learned demonology, had no place for *magia naturalis*, for the preternatural, for a middle ground between supernatural intervention, divine or demonic, and ordinary human manipulation of the natural world. The likeliest possibility was that Jeanne was a silly pretender – that is that she did not cure, the state of affairs that would perhaps best suit the faculty's claim to what we would now call a professional monopoly. But they could not exclude the possibility that she was something much worse – a non-physician who might sometimes cure her patients, yes; but also a witch in league with the devil.

We can see in this encounter a set of shared beliefs in, among other things, the possibility of witchcraft and miraculous healing, though defined in divergent ways. In the eyes of the physicians, if Jeanne actually claimed the latter, she was probably guilty of the former. A century later most physicians had renounced these beliefs. Prosecutions for the crime of witchcraft ended in 1682; a healer who boasted of miraculous powers might have been charged with swindling, but not with witchcraft. We can also see differences in medical practices. Despite the parallels one can find between some of Jeanne's remedies and those described in earlier writings by physicians, some of her therapies no longer made sense to the physicians, even though they made sense to Jeanne and her patients.

Conclusion

Although the sources are rarely rich enough to make it possible, microhistory of this kind is very useful for analyzing differences in health-related beliefs and practices where they are characterized by heterogeneity, eclecticism, and variability, and it is hard to identify contrasting coherent 'systems'.[84] As a generation of work on the history of the patient reminds us, we must pay attention to the individual as a historical subject, as she or he makes medical choices – the treatments accepted or refused, and the reasons for which a therapy appears credible (or not) – but also the encounters between practitioner and patient. Each encounter necessarily implies some points in common, without which communication would not be possible (as Brockliss and Jones emphasize), but also differences, which may possibly affect diagnosis and therapeutics. When

on 'Witchcraft and Popular Mentality in Lorraine, 1580–1630' concludes that 'the pact was clearly a part of popular belief' (p. 68) and minimizes distinctions between elite and popular views of witchcraft in this region.

84 For the use of 'heterogeneity', 'eclecticism', and 'variability', see Miles/Leatherman (2002).

the divergence is extreme, conflicts can arise. Highly focussed studies can also shed light on the interactions of individuals in small groups, such as Jeanne Lescallier and her supporters.

We do, however, need to generalize if we are to avoid the sort of pointillism that makes comparison and analysis impossible. In order to make meaningful generalizations, we need categories, whether they are based on Max Weber's ideal types, Wittgenstein's family resemblances or something else.[85] Out of what may seem to outsiders like disciplinary chauvinism, some historians despise sociology and anthropology and bar the use of models, typologies, and taxonomies. Such scepticism may run the risk of falling into a rather naive nominalism.[86] Citing examples and counter-examples to show that a model or category does not work does not suffice as a method. Categories are heuristic tools that we construct, according to the problems that we seek to address, rather than natural species all of whose members possess the same characteristics. For some purposes a distinction, say, between Galenic and non-Galenic therapies is useful and interesting. In the Lescallier case, the category of *devin-guérisseur* may be more helpful than not, depending in part, of course, on the trial testimony one believes.

Eclecticism does not exclude the possibility of identifying with others who share certain beliefs and feelings as oposed to those who do not. 'Medical subculture' is no doubt too strong; it implies too much internal coherence and too much differentiation among groups. It may be helpful to think, instead, of epistemic communities, not in the narrow sense in which the term has been used in political science – international teams of experts – but in the sense of groups sharing ways of knowing the world.[87] Such communities are unstable, have porous boundaries, and are continually engaged in exchanges and appropriations. The same individual can belong, at least potentially, to multiple communities, whose principles and beliefs are not always perfectly compatible or even internally consistent. Lescallier, self-proclaimed protégée of a great charitable lady, active empiric, and reputed village cunning woman, is a case in point.

Bibliography

Baer, Hans A.: Biomedicine and Alternative Healing Systems in America: Issues of Class, Race, Ethnicity and Gender. Madison, WI 2001.
Baer, Hans A.: Medical Pluralism: An Evolving and Contested Concept in Medical Anthropology. In: Singer, Merrill; Erickson, Pamela I. (eds.): A Companion to Medical Anthropology. Malden, MA; Chichester 2011, pp. 405–423.
Bailey, Kenneth D.: Typologies and Taxonomies: An Introduction to Classification Techniques. Thousand Oaks, CA 1994.
Beik, William: A Social and Cultural History of Early Modern France. Cambridge 2009.

85   See Bailey (1994).
86   See, for example, Lindemann (1992).
87   On the political science model, see Haas (1992).

Bell, David Avrom: The Cult of the Nation in France: Inventing Nationalism, 1680–1800. Cambridge, MA 2001.

Bivins, Roberta: Alternative Medicine? A History. Oxford 2007.

Bodin, Jean: La Démonomanie des sorciers. Paris 1587.

Bouteiller, Marcelle: La Médecine populaire d'hier et d'aujourd'hui. Paris 1966.

Bowness, Charles: The Romany Way to Health. London 1970.

Braudel, Fernand: The Identity of France. 2 vols. Translated by Sian Reynolds. London 1988–1990.

Briggs, Robin: Communities of Belief: Cultural and Social Tension in Early Modern France. Oxford 1989.

Brightman, Robert: Forget Culture: Replacement, Transcendence, Relexification. In: Cultural Anthropology 10 (1999), pp. 509–546.

Brockliss, Laurence; Jones, Colin: The Medical World of Early Modern France. Oxford 1997.

Broomhall, Susan: Women's Medical Work in Early Modern France. Manchester; New York 2004.

Brunschwig, Hieronymus: Dis ist das Buch der Cirurgia: Hantwirchung der Wundartzny. Strasbourg 1497.

Burke, Peter: Popular Culture in Early Modern Europe. New York 1978.

Burnham, John: What is Medical History? Cambridge 2005.

Cant, Sarah; Sharma, Ursula: A New Medical Pluralism? Alternative Medicine, Doctors, Patients, and the State. London 1999.

Carbonnier-Burkard, Marianne; Cabanel, Patrick: Une histoire des protestants en France, XVIe-XXe siècle. Paris 1998.

Choppin, René: De privilegiis rusticorum. Frankfurt/Main 1608.

Clark, Stuart: Thinking with Demons: The Idea of Witchcraft in Early Modern Europe. Oxford 1997.

Dunn, Frederick L.: Traditional Asian Medicine and Cosmopolitan Medicine as Adaptive Systems. In: Leslie, Charles M. (ed.): Asian Medical Systems. A Comparative Study. Berkeley 1976, pp. 133–158.

Ebrahimnejad, Hormoz (ed.): The Development of Modern Medicine in Non-Western Countries: Historical Perspectives. London 2009.

Ernst, Waltraud: Plural Medicine, Tradition and Modernity. Historical and Contemporary Perspectives: Views From Below and From Above. In: Ernst, Waltraud (ed.): Plural Medicine, Tradition and Modernity, 1800–2000. London; New York 2002, pp. 1–18.

Fadiman, Anne: The Spirit Catches You and You Fall Down: A Hmong Child, Her American Doctors, and the Collision of Two Cultures. New York 1997.

Garnier, André: Le Délit d'exercice illégal de la médecine. Paris 1937.

Gentilcore, David: From Bishop to Witch: The System of the Sacred in Early Modern Terra D'Otranto. Manchester 1992.

Gentilcore, David: Healers and Healing in Early Modern Italy. Manchester; New York 1998.

Gentilcore, David: Figurations and State Authority in Early Modern Italy: The Case of the Sienese Protomedicato. In: Canadian Journal of History 34 (1999), pp. 359–383.

Gentilcore, David: Was There A 'Popular Medicine' in Early Modern Europe? In: Folklore 115 (2004), pp. 151–166.

Gentilcore, David: Medical Charlatanism in Early Modern Italy. Oxford 2006.

Goldstein, Michael S.: The Persistence and Resurgence of Medical Pluralism. In: Journal of Health Politics, Policy and Law 29 (2004), pp. 925–945.

Goubert, Jean-Pierre: Malades et médecins en Bretagne, 1770–1790. Rennes 1974.

Guthrie, Douglas: A History of Medicine. Philadelphia; London; Montreal 1946.

Haas, Peter M.: Introduction: Epistemic Communities and International Policy Coordination. In: International Organization 46 (1992), pp. 1–35.

Henry, John: Doctors and Healers: Popular Culture and the Medical Profession. In: Pumfrey, Stephen; Rossi, Paolo L.; Slawinski, Maurice (eds.): Science, Culture and Popular Belief in Renaissance Europe. Manchester 1991, pp. 191–221.

Herzlich, Claudine: Patients, Practitioners, Social Scientists and the Multiple Logics of Caring and Healing. In: Jütte, Robert et al. (eds.): Historical Aspects of Unconventional Medicine: Approaches, Concepts, Case Studies. Sheffield 2001, pp. 27–36.

Jenner, Mark S. R.; Wallis, Patrick (eds.): Medicine and the Market in England and its Colonies, c.1450 – c.1850. Basingstoke 2007.

Jones, Colin: Medicine, Madness and Mayhem from the Roi Soleil to the Golden Age of Hysteria. In: French History 4 (1990), pp. 378–388.

Jones, Colin: The Cambridge Illustrated History of France. Cambridge 1994.

Jones, Colin: The Great Chain of Buying: Medical Advertisement, the Bourgeois Public Sphere and the Origins of the French Revolution. In: American Historical Review 101 (1996), pp. 13–40.

Joubert, Laurent: Erreurs populaires au fait de la medecine et regime de santé. Bordeaux 1578.

Joubert, Laurent: Segonde partie des Erreurs populaires, et propos vulgaires, touchant la medecine & le regime de santé Avec deus catalogues de plusieurs autres erreurs ou propos vulgaires, qui n'ont été mancionnés an la premiere & segonde edition de la premiere partie. Paris 1579.

Jütte, Robert: Alternative Medicine and Medico-Historical Semantics. In: Jütte, Robert; Eklöf, Motzi; Nelson, Marie C. (eds.): Historical Aspects of Unconventional Medicine: Approaches, Concepts, Case Studies. Sheffield 2001, pp. 11–23.

Kaptchuk, Ted J.; Eisenberg, David M.: Varieties of healing, 1: Medical Pluralism in the United States. In: Annals of Internal Medicine 135 (2001), pp. 189–195.

Kaptchuk, Ted J.; Eisenberg, David M.: Varieties of healing, 2: A Taxonomy of Unconventional Healing Practices. In: Annals of Internal Medicine 135 (2001), pp. 196–204.

Lancre, Pierre de: L'Incrédulité et mescréance du sortilège pleinement convaincue. Paris 1622.

Lanning, John Tate; TePaske, John Jay: The Royal Protomedicato. The Regulation of the Medical Professions in the Spanish Empire. Durham, NC 1985.

Last, Murray: Understanding Health. In: Skelton, Tracey; Allen, Tim (eds.): Culture and Global Change. London 1999, pp. 81–83.

Lecca, Pedro J. et al.: Cultural Competency in Health, Social, and Human Services: Directions for the Twenty-First Century. New York 1998.

Lémery, Nicolas: Dictionnaire ou traité universel des drogues simples [...]. 3rd ed. Amsterdam 1716.

Leslie, Charles M.: The Modernization of Asian Medical Systems. In: Poggie Jr., John; Lynch, Robert N. (eds.): Rethinking Modernization. Westport, CT 1974, pp. 69–108.

Leslie, Charles M. (ed.): Asian Medical Systems: A Comparative Study. Berkeley 1976.

Leslie, Charles M.: The Ambiguities of Medical Revivalism in Modern India. In: Leslie, Charles M. (ed.): Asian Medical Systems: A Comparative Study. Berkeley 1976, pp. 356–367.

LeVest, Barnabé: CCXXXVII Arrests célèbres et mémorables du parlement de Paris. Paris 1612.

Lindemann, Mary: Confessions of an Archive Junkie. In: Karsten, Peter; Modell, John (eds.): Theory, Method and Practice in Social and Cultural History. New York 1992, pp. 152–180.

Lindemann, Mary: Health & Healing in Eighteenth-Century Germany. Baltimore 1996.

Lindemann, Mary: Medicine and Society in Early Modern Europe. 2nd ed. Cambridge 2010.

Littlewood, Roland (ed.): On Knowing and Not Knowing in the Anthropology of Medicine. Walnut Creek, CA 2007.

López Terrada, María Luz: Medical Pluralism in the Iberian Kingdoms: The Control of Extra-Academic Practitioners in Valencia. In: Medical History Supplement 29 (2009), pp. 7–25.

Mandrou, Robert: Magistrats et sorciers en France au XVIIe siècle: Une analyse de psycholo-
    gie historique. Paris 1968.
Miles, Ann; Leatherman, Thomas: Perspectives on Medical Anthropology in the Andes. In:
    Koss-Chioino, Joan D.; Leatherman, Thomas; Greenway, Christine (eds.): Medical Plural-
    ism in the Andes. London 2002, pp. 6–7.
Muchembled, Robert: Popular Culture and Elite Culture in France, 1400–1750. Translated by
    Lydia Cochrane. Baton Rouge 1985.
Muchembled, Robert: Sorcières: justice et société aux 16e et 17e siècles. Paris 1987.
Perdiguero, Enric: El pluralisme mèdic: una clau interpretativa per a una història integral de
    la medicina. In: Ciencia e Ideología en la Ciudad. Vol. 2. Valencia 1994, pp. 211–227.
Pliny: Natural History. Translated by Harris Rackham. 10 vols. Cambridge, MA 1938–1963.
Pomata, Gianna: Contracting a Cure: Patients, Healers, and the Law in Early Modern Bolo-
    gna. Baltimore 1998.
Porcheron, Edgar-Jean-Ernest: Les Braconniers de la médecine au pays de Poitou. Bordeaux
    1923.
Porter, Roy: Before the Fringe: Quack Medicine in Georgian England. In: History Today 36
    (1986), pp. 16–22.
Porter, Roy: Before the Fringe: 'Quackery' and the Eighteenth-Century Medical Market. In
    Cooter, Roger (ed.): Studies in the History of Alternative Medicine. New York 1988, pp.
    1–27.
Porter, Roy: Quacks: Fakers and Charlatans in English Medicine. Stroud 2000.
Purnell, Larry D.; Paulanka, Betty J. (eds.): Transcultural Health Care: A Culturally Compe-
    tent Approach. Philadelphia 1998.
Ramsey, Matthew: Professional and Popular Medicine in France, 1770–1830: The Social
    World of Medical Practice. Cambridge 1988.
Ramsey, Matthew: Alternative Medicine in Modern France. In: Medical History 43 (1999),
    pp. 286–322.
Redfield, Robert: Peasant Society and Culture. An Anthropological Approach to Civilization.
    Chicago 1956.
Roelcke, Volker: Medikale Kultur: Möglichkeiten und Grenzen der Anwendung eines kultur-
    wissenschaftlichen Konzepts in der Medizingeschichte. In: Paul, Norbert; Schlich, Thomas
    (eds.): Medizingeschichte: Aufgaben, Probleme, Perspektiven. Frankfurt/Main 1998, pp.
    45–68.
Scheid, Volker; MacPherson, Hugh (eds.): Integrating East Asian Medicine into Contempo-
    rary Healthcare. Edinburgh 2012.
Sewell, William H., Jr.: The Concept(s) of Culture. In: Bonnell, Victoria E.; Hunt, Lynn (eds.):
    Beyond the Cultural Turn: New Directions in the Study of Society and Culture. Berkeley
    1999, pp. 35–61.
Shatzmiller, Joseph: Jews, Medicine, and Medieval Society. Berkeley 1994.
Starr, Paul: The Social Transformation of American Medicine. New York 1982.
Stein, Claudia: Negotiating the French Pox in Early Modern Germany. Farnham 2009.
Thomas, Keith: Religion and the Decline of Magic. London 1971.
Turgeon, Charles: Les Manuscrits de Simon Marion et la coutume de Paris au XVIe siècle. In:
    Travaux juridiques et économiques de l'Université de Rennes 8 (1923), pp. 135–157.
Villiers, A. de: Vieux procès angevins. In: Revue de l'Anjou N. S. 48 (1904), pp. 365–369.
Winnick, Terri A.: From Quackery to 'Complementary' Medicine: The American Medical
    Profession Confronts Alternative Therapies. In: Social Problems 52 (2005), pp. 38–61.
Zarzoso, Alfons: El pluralismo médico a través de la correspondencia privada en la Cataluña
    del siglo XVIII. In: Dynamis: Acta Hispanica ad Medicinae Scientiarumque Historiam
    Illustrandam 21 (2001), pp. 409–433.
Zimmels, Hirsch Jakob: Magicians, Theologians, and Doctors: Studies in Folk Medicine and
    Folklore as Reflected in the Rabbinical Responsa. Northvale, NJ 1997.

'The Diffusion of Useful Information': Household Practice, Domestic Medical Guides and Medical Pluralism in Nineteenth-Century Britain

Hilary Marland

Introduction

This article explores practices of plural medicine through the particular prism of medical advice literature intended for household use in nineteenth-century Britain.[1] Both orthodox and alternative systems of medicine offered guidance on the implementation of therapeutic techniques in domestic settings though household medical guides, which additionally provided detailed information on the prevention of disease, hygiene, regimen, responses to accidents, as well as advice targeted more specifically at women and children. The range of household guides increased, as volumes authored by 'orthodox' practitioners were supplemented by those produced by advocates of the new healing approaches that emerged during the nineteenth century, including hydropathy, homoeopathy and medical botany (or Thomsonianism). In varying degrees and in varying ways, all emphasised the possibilities of domestic interventions in health maintenance and therapy. Household medical guides – whatever their philosophical or therapeutic starting points – aimed at the 'diffusion of useful information', providing straightforward instructions on health maintenance and the treatment of mundane, everyday conditions, and many also gave advice on serious, even life-threatening conditions.[2] They were after all predominantly presented as 'medical' guides rather than guides to 'health'. It will be suggested here that guides on domestic medicine opened homes up to the possibilities of medical pluralism, advertised the array of medical systems on offer and the relative ease of annexing their recommendations in the home. However, it will also be suggested that while families or individuals attracted to domestic medicine may have held a strong allegiance to a particular set of medical theories or ideologies, in some respects household practice – and the guides advocating this – overrode differences between allopathic and competing systems of medicine in terms of their methodologies and attention to regimen and lifestyle.

---

1   There is a limited literature on domestic practices in nineteenth-century Britain, but for North America, see, for example, Murphy (1991) and Rosenberg (2003).
2   South (1852), preface to 2nd ed. 1849.

Domestic Medicine and the 'Active Patient' in Nineteenth-Century Britain

It is suggested here that rather than the nineteenth-century being a period of decline in terms of domestic practices of medicine, it witnessed their continued reinvention and even expansion, spurred by increased access to medical supplies and equipment, as well as new information resources intended to instruct 'active patients', patients keen to learn and apply techniques of healing or health improvement. Traditional domestic practices appear to have survived and were added to by the novel approaches of new systems of medicine, as well as the expansion in available medical supplies and the merchandising of equipment ranging from scales and measuring devices to inhalers, enema apparatus, ear douches and kit baths. These were marketed through local retailers, notably chemists and druggists, as well as newspapers, trade catalogues and via medical guides themselves, and given a further boost by new advertising techniques, including lavish printed illustrations and attractive shop displays.[3]

Domestic spaces were seen as appropriate loci of practice by those promoting orthodox, homoeopathic and hydropathic medical therapies, while the new system of medical botany introduced to England from North America by Samuel Thomson in the mid-nineteenth century, which was particularly influential in the industrial north, was at least in its early years directed towards healing practices centred in the home, with its intention of making 'every man his own doctor'.[4] Though the therapeutic approaches recommended could be – although were not necessarily – divergent, the emphasis on training patients to carry out simple procedures and to dose family members with straightforward remedies was shared by all those promoting domestic practices of medicine, although they varied in their content and the degree of checks and balances attached to their recommendations.

Exploration of the varied forms of print culture which grew in scope during this period – and became, by virtue of modest pricing in many cases, more accessible – notably household medical guides, pamphlets and lay health periodicals, offers insight into the ways in which text and material culture converged to provide 'toolkits' to equip patients eager to treat their family members or to prevent disease. The literature also became increasingly global, with health guides traversing between North America and Britain in particular.[5] The review pages of lay periodicals, meanwhile, provide insight into both laudatory and critical reception of household medicine texts. Tantalising evidence is offered by family recipe books, which continued to be compiled or added to in new hands throughout the century, demonstrating continued allegiance to self-healing and the practice of treating family, friends and neighbours. Recipe books also indicate the ways in which prescriptive literature in-

3   See Richards (1990), especially chapter 4 on patent medicines.
4   Pickstone (1976/77); Miley/Pickstone (1988); Marland (1987/2008), pp. 226–228.
5   Gevitz (1992).

formed and facilitated the making up of medical remedies in the home and practices of nursing, preventative health care, regimen and treatment. This article draws in particular on a sample of mid-nineteenth-century medical guides, to explore the methodologies and practices they advocated in the home, based on the assumption, supported by the continued production and sale of large numbers of these texts and the interest they stimulated in lay media, that homes contained potentially 'active patients' eager to take up this advice.

Exploration of domestic medicine in the nineteenth century enables us to envisage such practices, given the resort to new techniques, medicaments and means of knowledge transmission, as urging medical innovation and in some cases (such as the need for a particular piece of apparatus in the home) driving change, a factor often overlooked given history of medicine's overriding preoccupation with professional agendas and institutional sites in the modern period. Certainly the promotion of domestic practices was important in boosting the popularity of hydropathy, homoeopathy and medical botany. It also permits us to explore the continued role of domestic medicine beyond the early modern period, which, in recent years, largely through the interrogation of recipe book collections, has been claimed as the heyday of household medicine.[6]

What is certain is that the nineteenth-century household was a key site of medical activity, evidenced by the continued production of recipe books, compiled in wealthy and less well-to-do households, that drew on an ever widening range of authorities and contacts to compile their contents – family members and networks of friends and neighbours, magazines and newspapers, and a range of suppliers of medical goods and services, including medical practitioners and chemists and druggists.[7] A recipe book compiled by a 'Coventry housewife' during the late eighteenth and early nineteenth centuries, for instance, took recipes from the *Coventry Mercury*, as well as attributing them to local medical figures, direct familial contacts and durable authorities such as Nicholas Culpepper.[8] In the early nineteenth century local weaver James Woodhead of Netherthong, West Yorkshire, made up a recipe book containing almost forty remedies based on easily obtainable medicaments and herbs, as well as pre-prepared remedies such as Widow Welch's Pills, a well-known abortificient, and female pills, composed of iron, aloes and antimony. It is likely that Woodhead relied for many of his raw materials on the local druggists shop.[9] As the number of chemists and druggists continued to grow – rapidly in many urban communities – they advertised the extent to which

6   Leong (2008); Leong/Pennell (2007); Smith (1985); Stine (1996); Stobart (2008).
7   Archival and library collections contain significant numbers of nineteenth-century recipe books, notably the Wellcome Library recipe book collection, which has a total of nearly 300 volumes, a number of which date up to the late nineteenth century.
8   Wellcome Library: MS7366. Collection of medical, veterinary, culinary and household recipes, apparently compiled by a Coventry housewife, late 18th-early 19th century.
9   Kirklees District Archives: MS KC 190/1. Woodhead, J, Netherthong, recipe book, 1818.

they specialised in the compounding of family recipes, the sale of medicines and raw ingredients for making up remedies in the home, as well as retailing a growing range of apparatus and patent medicines for domestic use. Medicine chests, stocked with a variety of potions and medicaments, were a staple sales item, targeted at families with varied budgets, or specifically for ladies, as well as travellers, clergymen and missionaries.[10] For some chemists and druggists, the compilation of family remedies and the supply of ingredients for domestic use appear to have been a mainstay of their business, and many kept note-books of prescriptions specifically for this purpose. Chemist H. Wilcox's rec-ipe book, dated 1860, for instance, listed an enormous range of products for domestic use, including corn plasters, lip salve, toothpaste and cocoa, as well as household recipes for eye lotions, cough mixtures, rheumatic pills, stomach bitters, embrocation and 'rose nipple liniment'.[11]

While by the nineteenth century the marketplace quack was a figure in decline, he or she was replaced by a different type of itinerant who operated not from the marketplace but from local retailers or public houses, a signifier of the ways in which some forms of medical practice were moving out of pub-lic arenas into private spaces. There was also a significant increase in the re-tailing of special preparations and patent remedies via newspapers and trade directories as well as chemists and druggists, publicans, grocers, hairdressers, booksellers, and so on. Some, such as John Kaye's Worsdell's Pills, 'the most extensively established Family Medicine of the present day', sold in boxes costing between 1s 1½d to 4s 6d, were advertised specifically as household remedies to be kept in stock in case of illness.[12] Such preparations ranged from the local, such as Wakefield chemist G. B. Reinhardt's Balsam of Hore-hound, for curing coughs, colds, asthmas, declines and consumptions, to global brands such as Eno's and Beecham's pills, intended to build robust health.[13] Patent medicines have been described predominantly as emblem-atic of an increasingly active commerce in medicine as well as a source of anxiety for the medical profession.[14] Yet they can also be conceived as being representative of the 'commercial end' of household medical practices, one of several options on offer in terms of purchasing medicines and using them at home in a ready made form. The market in preparations for treating venereal diseases was particularly energetic from the eighteenth century onwards, as was the retail of 'female pills', indicating a more furtive aspect of household medical practice.[15]

10   Marland (2006).
11   Wellcome Library: MS8029. Chemist's recipe book, signed 'H. Wilcox 1860', compris-ing list of ingredients with quantities.
12   Marland (1987/2008), pp. 222–225, 243–244. For the retail of opiates, see Berridge (1987/1999).
13   Marland (1987/2008), p. 242; Ueyama (2010), p. 97.
14   Richards (1990); Loeb (2001); Ueyama (2010), chapter 2; Porter (1989), chapter 8.
15   Porter (1989), chapter 6; Elder (2007).

Household Medical Guides: Intent and Purpose

Household health manuals were vigorously marketed throughout the nineteenth century by medical practitioners and publishers, and its closing decades were marked by the production of a number of health periodicals targeted at a lay readership such as *Good Health* and *Domestic Health*.[16] Books and journals catering especially for women, such as *The British Mothers' Journal* and *The Mothers' Companion*, advised particularly on the health of married women and their infants and children.[17] The production of this vast array of medical guides was part of a wider expansion in advice literature which was becoming more secular in nature as well as being increasingly targeted at family audiences from the 1830s and 1840s onwards.[18] William Buchan's 'Domestic Medicine', first published in 1769, is far and away the best known of these; it sold over 80,000 copies in Buchan's lifetime (1729–1805) and new editions followed throughout the nineteenth century.[19] Numerous other health manuals offered detailed information and training to households, advising and supporting the medical activities of families in a range of circumstances.

Reviews in popular and literary periodicals indicate not only interest in these texts but also the continued vitality of domestic medical practice, though the reviews were far from being uniformly congratulatory on the quality of the texts or supportive of domestic interventions. A review of South's 'Household Surgery' described its purpose as 'alarming' and 'emphatically protested' against some of the procedures referred to in the book, including drawing teeth, cupping and reducing factures.[20] John Gardner was chastised for his focus on the cure of disease rather than its prevention following the publication of his 'Household Medicine'; anyone, noted the reviewer, who regarded the teaching of physiology as enabling the public to treat their own diseases was 'encouraging a delusion'.[21] Despite such negative reviews, medical authors including South and Gardner, as well as Richard Reece, Thomas Graham, John Savory and Spencer Thomson, enjoyed great popularity, in terms of the numbers of books produced and sold and their public exposure, while reviewers commented on the overthrow of one authority by another: 'Buchan's reign was once universal, [...] till Thomson hurled him from his throne; and Thomson [...] is pushed from his stool by Dr. Graham.'[22] Despite being hurled from his stool, Thomson's 'Dictionary of Domestic Medicine and Household Surgery' was still going strong several decades later; in 1882 the

16 See Rosenberg (2003), pp. 1–20.
17 For female readership of medical advice, see Flint (1993); for infant and child care, Branca (1975), chapter 6, and Petermann (2007).
18 Stearns/Stearns (1986), chapter 3.
19 Lawrence (1975). See also Porter (1985) for the impact of literary magazines on lay medical knowledge.
20 Anon. (1850).
21 Anon. (1861).
22 Anon. (1828).

twenty-forth edition, revised by J.C. Steele, assisted by Thomson, made its appearance, having been modernised and revised to include more material on preventive medicine.[23] South's 'Household Surgery', regarded as an early form of first aid manual, was reissued four times in the five years following its first publication in 1847.

Household medical guides set out to provide prospective patients with a toolkit of knowledge and information on the equipment and medicaments required to practice medicine in the home. They provided detailed lists of drugs and chemicals, explaining their actions and applications, as well as recommendations on the treatment of a vast array of diseases and disorders, from the mundane to the critical. Many, like John Savory's volume first published in 1836, provided explanations of weights, measures and dosages, as well as extensive lists of the equipment and medicaments required for domestic practice, shopping lists essentially of items to have in the home. Savory also explained how to make up gargles, infusions, eye lotions, clysters, liniment, and washes for venereal sores.[24] Additionally, household guides explained the techniques associated with medical interventions, minor surgery and preventative medicine, hygiene and regimen. They placed a great deal of emphasis on regimen as well as the constitutions, habits, and circumstances of their patients, which would entail different approaches to treatment and dosages: 'Women generally require smaller doses than men, and the state of their uterine functions should never be overlooked', Savory claimed, while 'Stimulants and purgatives more readily affect the sanguine than the phlegmatic'.[25]

Physician Richard Reece first published his 'Domestic Medical Guide' in 1803, which provided detailed instructions on how to furnish a family medical chest, item by item, listing all medicines, clearly numbered, and a precise guide to their properties and dosage.[26] Reece's focus in this volume was on guiding his readers through the use of fully fitted medicine chests, and he clearly anticipated that families would actively treat themselves, and required the wherewithal to do this in terms of knowledge on how to best utilise their purchases. Reece had a successful London practice and in addition studied chemistry and botany, and his knowledge of the properties of plants enabled him to introduce several new drugs into general use.[27] He placed great faith too in old remedies. Tincture of Rhubarb (No. 4 in his medical chest) was recommended as a purge in colicky and flatulent affections of the bowels, for weakness and laxity of the stomach and intestines and for a sluggish liver. No. 6 Compound Tincture of Senna was a further option for tackling colic and flatulence, while Reece made several recommendations involving combinations of ingredients from his medical chests for more specific disorders of the

23   Thomson [1882?].
24   Savory (1836).
25   Savory (1836), p. xii.
26   Reece (1803).
27   Power (2012).

digestive system.[28] Reece edited the *Monthly Gazette of Health* for many years, which had as its goal the diffusion of knowledge of medicine amongst wider publics.

The majority of domestic guides included statements on the intended usage and users of their volumes. John Savory's 'Compendium of Domestic Medicine' was directed at training family members,

> to enable unprofessional persons to obtain, at one glance, information regarding the effects and uses of the substances employed in medicine, and the mode of combining them for administration in the various diseases in which they have, by long experience, been found useful.

Savory employed his preface, as did many other authors, to promote his book above other domestic guides, which he castigated for their 'vague directions'. His work was also 'divested as much as possible of technical and scientific phraseology'. Savory, who was a Member of the Society of Apothecaries, went on, however, to warn that 'It is, however, earnestly recommended not to place too much confidence on books of Domestic Medicine, especially in such cases as are of a serious nature, but always have recourse to the advice of an able physician as early as it can be obtained'.[29] Despite this, his detailed guidance on weights and measures, doses and medical apparatus, appeared designed to equip readers with detailed knowledge and technical know-how.

Like many authors of domestic manuals, Savory specified that his guide was to be used with caution, and was intended for a specific audience, in Savory's case for

> travellers, and those humane characters who, residing at a distance from a duly qualified medical practitioner, devote a portion of their time to the relief and mitigation of the complicated misfortunes of disease and poverty among their poor neighbours.[30]

Jabez Hogg's domestic guide declared a similar intention of offering the best medical advice to persons residing at a distance from medical men in cases of sudden illness of accidents 'that such misfortunes may be alleviated, perhaps cured, but at any rate not rendered worse in the absence of professional aid'. However, he cautioned against the overuse of self-dosing:

> The person who purchases a stock of medicines and instructs himself to mix and make up drugs, must avoid giving way to a desire to practice his skill on every trivial occasion. He should only administer when the advice of a medical man is unattainable, and the case is imperative.[31]

Yet the volume offered advice on medicine and surgery not only for domestic use and use in the nursery, but also the 'cottage' and the 'bush', and contained remarkable detail on the practice of medicine and surgery for emigrants, travellers, missionaries and sea captains. It is hard to conceive that an interested household practitioner would be so obedient as to stop reading once they

28   Reece (1803), pp. 9, 11.
29   Savory (1836), pp. iii–iv.
30   Savory (1836), p. iv.
31   Hogg [1853?], p. vii.

reached the advice intended for those living in rural areas, on ships or on overseas missions.

Surgeon John Flint South's 'Household Surgery', first published in 1847, was directed in particular at villagers and local clergy, but by the fourth edition he declared that his little book was 'now on most folks' table'. South emphasised a pragmatic, practical approach to the task in hand of treating family members:

> As it is impossible for any workman to practise his craft without tools, so it is needful that the person who, for the nonce, is to occupy the place of the Surgeon, should have 'all appliances and means to boot', wherewith he may be enabled to employ his skill to the best advantage.[32]

South gave detailed directions on the making of poultices, washes, plasters, ointments, and 'other necessary things', his so-called 'Doctor's Shop', and provided a straightforward and comparatively brief list (others, like Savory's were much longer) of the basics required for household dosing and the treatment of accidents: linseed meal, poppy heads and camomile flowers for poultices and fomentations, plasters, soap, camphor and mustard for liniments, and so on. South embedded his advice very much in the day-to-day functioning of households where funds were limited, recommending linen and flannel for making rollers and bandages, cut up straw as a cheap filling for pillows, and recycled hat or bonnet boxes for making splints. A 'Doctor's Shop' need be neither expensive nor cumbrous; medicine chests were an unnecessarily luxury, except for those who were excessively neat or liked 'nicknacks'.

The authors of such guides were regular practitioners, with Reece, Savory and South being qualified respectively in the three branches of medicine as a physician, apothecary and surgeon, while Hogg specialised as an ophthalmic surgeon. At a time when the medical marketplace was becoming overstocked and increasingly competitive, it seems remarkable that these practitioners would imperil their practices by advocating the practice of medicine in the household, whatever limitations they may have placed on this. The publicity these guides generated for their authors, however, is likely to have been rich compensation, leading to more rather than less custom, while the actual income from the sale of volumes with large print runs was significant. In any case, at a time when medical men were guarding against being associated with the commerce of medicine and in particular advertising their practices, this form of self advertisement appears to have represented an opportunity rather than an impediment to successful practice. South, for example, based at Blackheath, then a village just outside of London, enjoyed much success in his London practice, and was lecturer, surgeon and governor to St Thomas's Hospital and a Fellow of the Linnean Society.[33]

Another clue to the motivation of these authors is provided by Spencer Thomson. He described his 'Dictionary of Domestic Medicine and Household

---

32 South (1852), p. 1.
33 Lindsey (2012).

Surgery' as constituting a bulwark against quackery. This was something Reece's 1828 'Medical Guide' also alluded to, his publications 'enabling the public to distinguish the man of merit from the pretender', which would ensure that domestic medicine would actually benefit 'men of science and experience'.[34] Thomson's work was intended, he declared, for

> people of moderate means – who, so far as medical attendance is concerned, are worse off than the pauper – who will not call in and fee their medical advisor for every slight matter, and in the absence of a little knowledge, *will* have recourse to the prescribing druggist, or to the patent quackery which flourishes upon ignorance.[35]

This idea of equipping the working man with medical knowledge was reiterated in Black's 'Household Medicine', published in 1883, who described how 'to the labouring classes the subject is of special importance, for health is the capital of the working man'. Though Black advised resort to a professional, when no medical help was at hand 'they must run the risk of prescribing for themselves'.[36] Surgeon, writer on sport, expert on dog breeding, editor of the *Provincial Medical and Surgical Journal*, and author of 'Domestic Medicine and Surgery' and several other advice books, J. H. Walsh [pseud. 'Stonehenge'], elucidated on the ways in which the production of medical guides could minimise risk.[37] He accepted that people would always treat themselves; providing them with a little knowledge and advice would at least improve their practices and make them less dangerous to themselves and their households. His book was simply intended to make 'dabblers in physic' more efficient.

> It is not, therefore, with a view of increasing the number of those who administer physic to themselves or their friends that this book is written, but rather in the hope that, if the practice is adopted by them, advantage may be taken of the information contained within it, which is offered in such a form that they may avail themselves of it with some hope of success, and without any great risk of doing mischief.[38]

'Alternative' Domestic Guides: 'Alternative' Approaches?

A large number of household manuals were produced by those advocating the new systems of medicine that emerged during the mid-nineteenth century. The prefaces to these volumes and their framing of a potential readership tended to differ significantly from those of the orthodox medical guides outlined above. Freer from the complicated justifications resulting from anxieties about the proper limits of domestic practice, the guides produced by homoeopathic and hydropathic practitioners and medical botanists focused much more on promoting these novel approaches to treatment and aimed to reach as wide an audience of potential users as possible. Yet, they too advised some

34   Reece (1828), p. 4
35   Thomson [1882?], p. viii. Emphasis in original.
36   Black (1883), p. 1.
37   Boase (2012).
38   Walsh (1875), p. iii.

degree of caution, and recommended the advantages of turning to an experienced practitioner in severe cases or to acquire sound advice on how to proceed with treatments.

Foremost amongst these new systems was hydropathy, based largely on imbibing large quantities of water, combined with its external application, by means of baths and douches, wet bandages and sheets, which gained in vogue in Britain in the early 1840s. While centred around treatments at a growing number of hydropathic establishments, hydropathy emphasised a key role for domestic healing, and aimed to extend the benefits of pure water, and advice on regimen, diet, exercise, clothing and lifestyle to those who could not afford to visit costly hydros.[39] As Joseph Constantine, a woollen weaver turned hydropathist who practised in the unlikely setting of industrial Manchester (thus refuting the need for scenic locations and costly lodgings to implement the water cure), declared in 1869 'Hydropathy is now spreading so rapidly that information of its principles and practices is required in the cottage as well as the mansion'.[40] The American health reformer and journalist Thomas Low Nichols declared that 'almost all the advantages and blessings of the water cure may be enjoyed at home, and that far cheaper, as a general thing, than any other system of medical treatment'. He offered tips on how to improvise cut-price bathing equipment: a tinman, cooper or carpenter could make a bath; oil cloth would protect carpets; and to have a thorough bath, a gallon of water was deemed sufficient. All that was required was air, exercise and proper food, 'All the rest is water, which can be had wherever rain falls, springs bubble, or rivers run'. 'The beauty of domestic hydropathy is that it is costless, open and free to all'.[41] Nichols emphasised that visitors to hydros represented merely the tip of a very large iceberg, the base of which was comprised of domestic users of hydropathy.

Hydropathists urged those visiting hydros for treatment to avail themselves of the training on offer there and to familiarise themselves with treatments which they could then continue at home, a practice most notably associated with Charles Darwin's exploits with the water cure; following visits to Malvern, he built an outdoor douche and bath in his garden and used these facilities daily for five years.[42] A number of hydropathic manuals were produced with the domestic market in mind, while hydropathic journals contained advice and information on techniques of water curing as well as accounts of the successful implementation of hydropathy in the home. John Smedley, proprietor of the vast Matlock Hydro in Derbyshire, and a man keen through his charitable Free Hospital to extend hydropathy to those of limited means, expounded the benefits of home treatments in his 'Practical Hydropathy', with a particular emphasis on making the system available to working people:

39   Marland/Adams (2009).
40   Constantine (1869), preface.
41   Nichols (1887), pp. 354, 415–416.
42   Browne (1990).

> One of the principle objects I have in view in this work is to teach Hydropathic remedies for self-application, and to show the labouring classes how to manage many of the processes by the simple means within their reach, which, if acted upon, would often stay the progress of fever, consumption, and inflammation, or prevent their proceeding beyond the first symptoms. Resolution, and not sparing trouble, alone are necessary.[43]

Hydropathists trod a fine line between wishing to advertise the merits of treatment at a dedicated hydropathic establishment and boosting their own practices and the possibilities of making the system accessible to all. The sale of products and manuals undoubtedly became a robust income stream for the several of the more successful hydropathists. At the same time as making stirring proclamations, as noted above, on the cheapness and accessibility of hydropathy, Nichols retailed costly and elaborate bathing equipment as well as foodstuffs via his journal, the *Herald of Health*. Smedley too sold a range of goods intended for domestic use, including kit form baths and other bathing equipment, foodstuffs, and clothing. Meanwhile, his book 'Practical Hydropathy' became something of a medical best seller; first published in 1858, by 1872 it had sold some 85,000 copies. His wife, Caroline's guide for women, meanwhile, went through fifteen editions between its first issue in 1861 and 1873, by which time it had sold 45,000 copies.[44] Both volumes, as well as being replete with advice on curing and preventative health measures, contained inspirational material in the form of letters of appreciation from those attempting to implement hydropathic techniques in the home and accounts of successful cures. One man, following Caroline Smedley's instructions, wrote of curing his wife's knee with applications of water – 'I paid every attention to your directions; and, bad as it was, I have made a perfect cure'.[45]

A striking feature of these guides is the fact that, while promoting their own systems of healing, some did not denounce allopathy altogether. Many combined a variety of approaches to healing – and thus advocated a plurality of practices – their pages including information on homoeopathy, hydropathy and general hygiene, as well as anatomy and physiology. As Pulte and Epps put it in their domestic guide to homoeopathy: 'These branches and parts of medical science [...] when properly understood and digested by the people, will, in a great degree, aid in augmenting the salutary results derivable from the use of a domestic physician'.[46] Nonetheless, the approach in their volume was founded on the careful selection of the correct homoeopathic remedy, and, given the importance of purity and careful adherence to the principle of diluting remedies, they strongly suggested that home users procured their medicine-chests from reliable sources, and should avoid chemists who sold old school medicines or who sold 'prostituted' 'homoeopathic tea' or 'homoeopathic coffee', etc.[47] Laurie's 'Homoeopathic Domestic Medicine' particu-

---

43 John Smedley (1861), p. xiv.
44 Rees (1988), p. 34; Caroline Smedley (1873).
45 Caroline Smedley (1880), p. 54.
46 Pulte/Epps (1859), p. vii.
47 Pulte/Epps (1859), p. 3.

larly recommended procuring medicine chests and medicines from A. C.
Clifton, a homoeopathic chemist of Northampton.[48] Edward Johnson published his 'Domestic Practice of Hydropathy' in 1849, with its declared objective of bringing the benefits of hydropathy within reach of the poor. An allo-
path by training before converting to hydropathy, Johnson saw hydropathy,
not as in opposition to allopathy, but 'complementary', and also stressed, as
did the writers of many domestic guides whatever their affiliation to a particular system of healing, that people would treat themselves at home 'whether
hydropathic physicians desire it or not' and that even an imperfect domestic
guide would be a valuable tool.[49] Edward Ruddock emphasised his belief that
there was much to learn from allopathic practitioners, and though 'Homoeopathy is the foundation on which his medical treatment is reared, he accepts
suggestions and profits by the experiences of others whenever and wherever
honestly presented'. He also stressed that his work was not intended to super-
sede homoeopathic treatment by experienced practitioners when it was accessible, but, somewhat in contradiction to his above statement, 'to recommend
remedies and measures of greater value and less dangerous, than those commonly employed in allopathic practice'.[50]

We can trace similarities in the pitches taken by authors of domestic guides
whatever their medical affiliation. They were keen not to blight their own
practices or to diminish their emphasis on the skills and reputation of experienced practitioners, but at the same time expressed the desire to make accessible good medical advice to those who lived at a distance from medical care
or who were unable to afford regular medical attention. They united in claim-
ing that good advice was a bulwark against households falling prey to poor
quality care or fraudulent practice, though allopaths were more likely to stand
in opposition to what they broadly construed as 'quackery' or the attentions of
prescribing chemists. Adherents of homoeopathy or hydropathy to varying
degrees saw themselves as offering an alternative to allopathic approaches,
involving less risky and less interventionalist methods of treatment. Hydopa-
thists eschewed the drug-based heroic methods of allopathic medicine in favour of the gentle healing effects of water, arguing that adherence to their
system put the patient in the best possible position to fight disease. Of the
medical 'alternatives', medical botany stands out in part for its close association with working-class politics, the temperance movement, vegetarianism
and Methodism (though other systems such as hydropathy shared some of
these allegiances), but more significantly for its resolute opposition to allopathic medicine and its practitioners. Medical botanists delighted in pointing
out divergences in methods of treatment on the part of regularly-qualified
medical men, which stood in sharp contrast to the unity of their approach,
destined to 'revolutionize the whole medical world'.[51] The techniques of med-

48   Laurie (1851).
49   Johnson (1848), pp. vi, ix–x.
50   Ruddock (1883), pp. 5–6.
51   Fox (1887), p. 10.

ical botany, based largely on Lobelia inflata, an emetic, and cayenne pepper, a counter-irritant and gastric stimulant, combined with the administration of herb teas, warmth and a nutritious diet, were regarded, in contrast to the mysteries of orthodox medicine, as empirical, natural, easy to comprehend and apply and effective.

Methodologies of Practice

Domestic guides – whatever their allegiance – stressed that there were limits to what should be attempted at home, and advised patients to seek professional or expert advice from an experienced practitioner in the case of serious disorders. In practice, however, they presented an impressive, and seemingly inexhaustible, array of disorders that could be treated in the confines of the home. Few, however, enlightened the reading public on what to do in the case of conditions that were difficult to diagnose, leaving a large grey area of uncertainty for domestic practitioners. The well-known Malvern hydopathist Dr James Gully placed 'a prudent limitation' on the number and character of conditions 'which I believe a usually educated and intelligent person may safely and efficiently venture to treat'.[52] However his 'Domestic Hydrotherapeia' went on to explain how to deal with fevers, coughs, indigestion, headaches, piles, rheumatism, brain fever and palpitations of the heart. Pulte and Epps' domestic homoeopathic guide, while advising expert intervention in its preface, offered detailed guidance on 'general diseases', largely chronic disorders or conditions related to general tiredness, overstrain and poor health – including lethargy, mental exhaustion, sleeplessness and sweating feet. It also provided information on how to treat fevers, affections of the head and mind, diseases of the eye, ear, face, nose and mouth, disorders of the stomach and bowels, windpipe and chest, the urinary and genital organs, the diseases of females and children and accidents – cholera, syphilis, phthisis and cancers were all included – rejecting few areas as being too ambitious for a household armed with their guide and a good quality medical chest. So too the domestic guides produced from early in the nineteenth century by regular doctors such as Reece and Graham had a similarly broad remit, providing guidance on disorders ranging from the mundane to deadly, which could involve the use of a potent set of drugs. Graham included, for example, advice on how to deal with attacks of epilepsy, not just the immediate paroxysms, but also its longer term management, providing information on new and innovative approaches, medical galvanism and external applications of opium: 'Though much cannot be said in favour of either of these remedies, yet, when other means fail of success, we may with propriety make a trial of them.'[53] Reece's guide included instruction on the use of laudanum (no. 18 in his medicine chest) for disease, the treatment of fevers, bowel disorders, and pain relief:

52 Gully (1863), pp. vi–vii.
53 Graham (1837), p. 409.

> When judiciously administered, this is, no doubt, the most valuable medicine in the whole *material medica*, and in certain stages, and with certain combinations, is advantageously employed in every disease incident to the human frame. It mitigates pain, induces sleep, allays inordinate action, and diminishes morbid irritability; hence it becomes an invaluable remedy in obviating and moderating symptomatic fevers from accidents. In spasmodic colic, it prevents inflammation of the bowels [...] In incurable diseases, where the sufferings of the patient are most excruciating, as in cancer &c. it wonderfully alleviates the miseries, and renders the life of the patient tolerable.[54]

What Reece did not allude to was the ease with which laudanum users slipped into addiction, though he did give advice on avoiding overdose as well as correcting the impact of laudanum on the digestive system.

While hydropaths, homoeopaths and medical botanists were similarly ambitious in terms of the disorders covered in their guides, their therapeutic approaches were of course very different to those of orthodox practitioners. Fox's 'Family Botanic Guide' decried the use of 'poisons', the lancet or cupping glass, 'and the use of that formidable enemy – the sheet anchor, the Goliath of medicine – that all-potent remedial agent of the medical profession [...] Mercury is altogether repudiated by the author'.[55] Hydropath Dr James Gully, himself trained in the allopathic system, but also one of its sternest critics, lambasted orthodox doctors for their indiscriminate use of drugs and local treatments, including bleeding, cauterisation and injections, remarking particularly on the plight of women patients subjected to these treatments which were often based on trumped up diagnosis for exploitation and profit.[56] Such opposition was most likely to be framed in terms of opposition to allopathic practitioners and orthodox medicine more generally rather than the domestic guides they authored.

When we turn to preventative approaches, however, a more unified picture emerges, certainly in the suggestion that prevention should prevail as being far more effective than curing. The majority of guides emphasised the role of lifestyle and regimen, and, while Edward Johnson argued that the chief advantage of hydropathy was that it put the body in 'the most favourable circumstances to resist and cure disease', domestic guides, whatever their therapeutic underpinning, devoted a good deal of attention to the subject of preventing disease.[57] Dr Jabez Hogg, an ophthalmic surgeon with attachments to several London hospitals, declared in his domestic guide, that medicine was an evil to be shunned, and in its place recommended attention to diet, ablutions, abstinence, air, clothing and exercise.[58] Bathing was advocated for a host of disorders or the boosting of general health, whether by hydropathists, homoeopathists, medical botanists or allopathic practitioners. Homoeopathist Edward Ruddock recommended the use of the bidet or hip bath to banish the

---

54   Reece (1828), pp. 23–24.
55   Fox (1887), preface.
56   Gully (1863), pp. 181–186, 219–238.
57   Johnson (1843), p. 70.
58   Hogg [1853?].

nervous, fancied, and real ailments of invalids, to provide relief for skin disorders and excessive sensitivity to cold, adding that

> Probably there is no hygienic habit inculcated in this volume commensurate in value to the cold bath; and although it is much neglected by the illiterate and poor, we are glad to know that it is now largely and increasingly adopted by the intelligent and well-to-do classes.[59]

Sheffield medical botanist William Fox urged the use of vapour or Turkish baths in his 'Family Botanic Guide'. Combined with stimulants and Lobelia inflata (one of the bedrocks of the botanic system),

> we have been able to cure tetanus or lockjaw in less than half an hour in every case; it is by the same means we have broken up the most obstinate cases of fever, which have baffled the most eminent physicians. And what we have done others can accomplish, if they will but attend to the laws of life, health, disease and its cure.[60]

By the 1860s James Gully was explaining that the hydropathic system was moving into 'ordinary practice':

> we hear of compresses being recommended by the better orders of the profession; we hear of *sitz* baths being ordered as an essential part of treatment; latterly we even hear of the learned Professors of the Practice of Physic in my own loved and revered University of Edinburgh packing patients suffering from scarlet fever in cold wet sheets.[61]

Dr Thomas Graham devoted many pages of his 'Modern Domestic Medicine' to the various techniques of bathing, cold, warm, tepid, vapour, as well as to bathing establishments and centres, and the benefits to be derived from imbibing mineral waters. He recommended vapour baths for a wide range of conditions, all cases of internal inflammation (since it draws blood to the surface and relieved the internal parts by the secretion of the skin), including fevers, inflammation of the bowels, stomach, etc., liver complaints, dropsy, obstinate rheumatic attacks, scrofulous and glandular swellings, gravel, palsy, and gout.[62] Graham also devoted a great deal of attention to diet, air, exercise, sleep, clothing and the passions; the latter he identified as a significant cause of disease. Though Thomson's 'Dictionary of Domestic Medicine', first published in 1852, consigned, 'unlicensed followers of the bi-millionth part of a billionth globule, or the marshy ways of water advocates [...] to a *terra incognita*', he emphasised the role of hygiene in improving both the health of individuals and the community, and recognised the value of the vegetarian diet and temperance, water being 'the only wholesome, *regular* drink of healthy men'.[63]

59 Ruddock (1883), p. 4.
60 Fox (1887), p. 93.
61 Gully (1863), pp. xi, ix. Emphasis in original.
62 Graham (1837), pp. 138–157, quote on p. 151.
63 Anon. (1853), quote on p. 90. Emphases in original.

Conclusion

In terms of methodology, domestic guides were keen to stress that patience and determination were essential parts of home practice. Approach and attitude was deemed important by those recommending domestic treatments across the board. Just as John Smedley had emphasised that 'Resolution, and not sparing trouble, alone are necessary',[64] Thomas Graham's guide promised 'to lay before his readers the best and most manageable remedies for the relief of pain and irritation, and the cure of disease', and also cautioned that perseverance was vital and that recovery was generally slow. 'In the practice of medicine, small beginnings frequently ripen into grand results, and it is too often from a disregard of this truth, and a foolish desire to try new plans of treatment, that persons afflicted with severe diseases fail to get well.'[65]

It is one thing to purchase a text; another to read it or actively employ it. We have, however, evidence of multiple editions, large print runs and the continued production of new domestic medical manuals throughout the nineteenth century, to suggest that they remained relevant. Certainly a market was perceived to exist. Charles Rosenberg has argued that

> It is no accident that so many popular health books survive in shabby condition, with recipes written on flyleaves or expanded with newspaper clippings recording cures for arthritis, consumption, or liver ailments. These books were not just read; they were used.[66]

Most household guides in my own modest collection have their owners' names written in the frontispiece and many are annotated, though this might indicate that they were regularly browsed rather than used actively as guides to treatment. In 1884 an 'Old Practitioner' while expressing some reservations about the benefits of household practice, urged that 'the practice of domestic medicine and the virtues which go with it long continue in our midst, and let no man be so ill-advised as to banish the harmless little medicine-chest with its associations from his hearth'.[67] A review of Black's 'Household Medicine', published in 1883, concluded that books on 'household medicine' were in great demand, as people were inspired – rather than discouraged – by the extension of scientific knowledge to be their own doctors.[68]

Exploration of domestic practices of medicine during the nineteenth century offers the opportunity to envisage the household as a site of both health promotion and treatment as well as the locus of practice of a variety of therapeutic approaches which allowed medical pluralism to exist and even flourish in this particular context. Medical interventions and practices of health within the home may have been driven by pragmatism, access and ideas of efficacy as well as by ideological and therapeutic support for orthodox or alternative

64   John Smedley (1861), p. xiv.
65   Graham (1837), pp. vi–vii.
66   Rosenberg (2003), p. 2.
67   By an Old Practitioner (1884), quote on p. 301.
68   Anon. (1883).

medicine, despite the missionary zeal which accompanied some systems and their firm stance in opposition to orthodox approaches. What is difficult to assess is the extent to which patients may have combined systems and adopted medical pluralism in the home, but the fact that many guides did this too is indicative of a range of approaches borrowing from different forms of practice; notably hydropathy and homoeopathy were commonly twinned at least in domestic contexts. Self-medicators, meanwhile, such as the naturalist and traveller Charles Waterton, Squire of Walton Hall, near Wakefield, drew on a variety of local expertise, including in his case bonesetters, as well as self-dosing; according to one source, Waterton bled himself on 136 occasions. He recommended fasting, and also developed his own prescriptions, including Mr Waterton's Pill, which was famed in his locality, and a powder for treating cases of cholera.[69] Though exceptionally adventurous in many ways, Waterton's curiosity about different approaches to medicine was reflected in the continued compilation of recipe books by many households and individuals throughout the nineteenth century, many of which drew on the knowledge and guidance contained in domestic guides.

The nineteenth century saw not only the burgeoning production of new means of promoting medical knowledge to the interested lay reader, but also the continuous adaptation of older, enduring forms of health transmission and the exchange of medical ideas, tips and remedies. In terms of medical pluralism, they involved not only the invocation of different systems of healing, but also resort to traditional and novel, even experimental, forms of practice. The nineteenth-century recipe book embodied both trends, with its compilers apparently eager to learn about and locate remedies from a variety of sources. Charlotte Hobhouse, who compiled her recipe book between 1824 and 1867, extracted recipes from newspapers and other printed sources which she glued in alongside handwritten recipes. She attributed remedies to the authors of well-known household guides, such as Dr Graham, as well as leading medical figures, including the surgeon Sir Astley Cooper. Some of her recipes were taken from London chemists or *The Times*, others from accounts of overseas travel or correspondence, such as Walpole's recommendation of alum to strengthen teeth or a recipe for marsh fever taken from a visitor's guide to Buffalo.[70]

Domestic practice appears to have allowed for some kind of cross over between systems of medicine, particularly in terms of methodology and approaches to healing and ideas of regimen, representing medical pluralism in a particularly fluid form. Domestic practice is likely too to have appealed to the public in terms of its adaptability and cost, though many domestic guides urged reliance on the purchase of elaborate equipment or a wide range of drugs to establish a doctors' shop at home and these were certainly not cheap

---

69   Marland (1987/2008), pp. 214–215, 221–222.
70   Wellcome Library: MS6826. Medical Recipe Book: A commonplace book of medical recipes, including pasted-in prescriptions and newspaper cuttings. The author, supposed to be Charlotte Hobhouse (1831–1914).

options. And while domestic medicine was apparently enduring, and often-times likely to have overridden considerations separating allopathy from its rivals, it also served to popularise new systems of medicine. Commenting upon the popularity of domestic medicine in general and homoeopathy in particular, Pulte and Epps explained how the first 'domestic physicians' were 'hailed' by the people in general

> as welcome friends in their domestic afflictions [...]. Imperfect as the first efforts of this kind naturally must have been, their beneficial results for families, and for the spread of Homoeopathy, were such that the improvement of these necessary medical guides were rapidly undertaken and accomplished.[71]

Much more inquiry is required to interrogate in detail what approaches active patients may have adopted in the home, and to understand what they might have thought about 'pluralistic' or complementary practices (if they considered this distinction at all). However, it is likely that a variety of medical systems flourished – stimulated by tradition and novelty, familiarity and new commercial drives – in a variety of domestic settings throughout the nineteenth century.

Bibliography

Anon.: Review of: Modern Domestic Medicine. By T.J. Graham, MD. In: Monthly Magazine, or British Register 6 (1828), no. 32 (August), p. 200.

Anon.: Review of: Hints on Emergencies. In: Household Words 2 (1850), no. 28 (5 October), pp. 47–48.

Anon.: Review: Thomson, Spencer. A Dictionary of Domestic Medicine and Household Surgery. In: Scottish Review 1 (1853), no. 1, pp. 89–91.

Anon.: Review of: Household Medicine; containing a Familiar Description of Diseases. By John Gardner, MD. In: The Atheneum 1774 (26 October 1861), p. 546.

Anon.: Medical Books. In: The Athenaeum 2883 (27 January 1883), pp. 122–123.

Berridge, Virginia: Opium and the People: Opiate Use and Drug Control Policy in Nineteenth and Early Twentieth Century England. Revised ed. London; New York 1999 [1st published 1987].

Black, George: Household Medicine: A Guide to Good Health, Long Life, and the Proper Treatment of all Diseases and Accidents. London 1883.

Boase, G.C. (revised Lock, Julian): Walsh, John Henry [pseud. Stonehenge] (1810–1888). In: Dictionary of National Biography, available at http://www.oxforddnb.com (accessed 12 Dec. 2012).

Branca, Patricia: Silent Sisterhood: Middle-Class Women in the Victorian Home. London 1975.

Browne, Janet: Spas and Sensibilities: Darwin at Malvern. In: Porter, Roy (ed.): The Medical History of Waters and Spas. Supplement 10 to Medical History. London 1990, pp. 102–113.

By an Old Practitioner (Anon.): Common Errors in Domestic Medicine. In: Chambers Journal 1 (1884), no. 19 (10 May), pp. 299–301.

---

71 Pulte/Epps (1859), p. vi.

Constantine, Joseph: Hydropathy at Home, or a Familiar Exposition of the Principles and Practice of the Water Cure. With Full Instructions for the Treatment of Diseases, Affections, Casualties, etc. London 1869.

Elder, Rachel: Rethinking Remedies for Women: Consumption, Regulation, and 'Female Pills', 1850–1914. Unpublished MA thesis, University of Warwick 2007.

Flint, Karen: The Woman Reader, 1837–1914. Oxford 1993.

Fox, William: The Working Man's Model Family Botanic Guide or Every Man his Own Doctor: Being an Exposition of the Botanic System, Giving a Clear and Explicit Explanation of the Botanic Practice, the Cause, Cure, and Prevention of Disease. 11th ed. Sheffield 1887.

Gevitz, Norman: 'But all those authors are foreigners': American Literary Nationalism and Domestic Medical Guides. In: Porter, Roy (ed.): The Popularization of Medicine 1650–1850. London 1992, pp. 232–251.

Graham, Thomas John: Modern Domestic Medicine: A Popular Treatise. 7th ed. London 1837.

Gully, James, MD: A Guide to Domestic Hydrotherapeia: The Water Cure in Acute Disease. London 1863.

Hogg, Jabez: The Domestic Medical and Surgical Guide, for the Nursery, the Cottage, and the Bush; Giving the Best Advice in the Absence of a Physician or Surgeon, in Cases of Sudden Illness: Useful to Families, Emigrants, Travellers, Missionaries, Village Clergymen, and Sea Captains. London [1853?].

Johnson, Edward: Hydropathy: The Theory, Principles, and Practice of the Water Cure Shewn to be in Accordance with Medical Science and the Teachings of Common Sense. London 1843.

Johnson, Edward: The Domestic Practice of Hydropathy. London 1848.

Laurie, J., MD: An Epitome of the Homoeopathic Domestic Medicine, Intended to Serve as a Guide to those who are Desirous of Commencing the Homoeopathic Treatment in Family Practice. London 1851.

Lawrence, C.J.: William Buchan: Medicine Laid Open. In: Medical History 19 (1975), pp. 20–35.

Leong, Elaine; Pennell, Sara: Recipe Collection and the Currency of Medical Knowledge in the Early Modern 'Medical Marketplace'. In: Jenner, Mark; Wallis, Patrick (eds.): Medicine and the Market in England and Its Colonies c.1450–1850. Houndmills 2007, pp. 133–152.

Leong, Elaine: Making Medicines in the Early Modern Household. In: Bulletin of the History of Medicine 82 (2008), pp. 145–168.

Lindsey, Christopher F.: South, John Flint (1797–1882). In: Dictionary of National Biography, available at http://www.oxforddnb.com (accessed 12 Dec. 2012).

Loeb, Lori: Doctors and Patent Medicine in Modern Britain: Professionalism and Consumerism. In: Albion. A Quarterly Journal Concerned with British Studies 33 (2001), pp. 404–425.

Marland, Hilary: Medicine and Society in Wakefield and Huddersfield 1780–1870. Cambridge 2008 [1st published 1987].

Marland, Hilary: 'The Doctor's Shop': The Rise of the Chemist and Druggist in Nineteenth-Century Manufacturing Districts. In: Hill, Louise (ed.): From Physick to Pharmacology: Five Hundred Years of British Drug Retailing. Aldershot 2006, pp. 79–104.

Marland, Hilary; Adams, Jane: Hydropathy at Home: The Water Cure and Domestic Healing in Mid-Nineteenth-Century Britain. In: Bulletin of the History of Medicine 83 (2009), pp. 499–529.

Miley, Ursula; Pickstone, J.V.: Medical Botany around 1850: American Medicine in Industrial Britain. In: Cooter, Roger (ed.): Studies in the History of Alternative Medicine. Houndmills 1988, pp. 140–154.

Murphy, Lamar Riley: Enter the Physician: The Transformation of Domestic Medicine, 1760–1860. Tuscaloosa; London 1991.

Nichols, Thomas Low: Nichols' Health Manual: Being Also a Memorial of the Life and Work of Mrs. Mary S. Gove Nichols. London 1887.

Petermann, Lisa: From a Cough to a Coffin: The Child's Medical Experience in Britain and France, 1762–1884. Unpublished PhD thesis, University of Warwick 2007.

Pickstone, J. V.: Medical Botany (Self-Help Medicine in Victorian England). In: Memoirs of the Manchester Literary and Philosophical Society 119 (1976/77), pp. 85–95.

Porter, Roy: Laymen, Doctors and Medical Knowledge in the Eighteenth Century: The Evidence of the Gentleman's Magazine. In: Porter, Roy (ed.): Patients and Practitioners. London 1985, pp. 138–168.

Porter, Roy: Health for Sale: Quackery in England 1660–1850. Manchester; New York 1989.

Power, D'Arcy (revised by Bevan, Michael): Reece, Richard (1775–1831). In: Dictionary of National Biography, available at http://www.oxforddnb.com (accessed 12 Dec. 2012).

Pulte, J. H.; Epps, John: Homoeopathic Domestic Physician. 5th ed. London 1859.

Reece, Richard: The Domestic Medical Guide; or, Complete Companion to the Family Medicine Chest. London 1803.

Reece, Richard: The Medical Guide. London 1828.

Rees, Kelvin: Water as a Commodity: Hydropathy in Matlock. In: Cooter, Roger (ed.): Studies in the History of Alternative Medicine. Houndmills 1988, pp. 28–45.

Richards, Thomas: The Commodity Culture of Victorian England: Advertising and Spectacle, 1851–1914. Stanford, CA 1990.

Rosenberg, Charles E. (ed.): Right Living: An Anglo-American Tradition of Self-Help Medicine and Hygiene. Baltimore; London 2003.

Ruddock, Edward: The Lady's Manual of Homoeopathic Treatment in the Various Derangements Incident to her Sex. 8th ed. London 1883.

Savory, John: A Compendium of Domestic Medicine: and Companion to the Medicine Chest. London 1836.

Smedley, Caroline: Ladies' Manual of Practical Hydropathy. 15th ed. London 1873.

Smedley, Caroline: Ladies' Manual of Practical Hydropathy. 19th ed. London 1880.

Smedley, John: Practical Hydropathy. 4th ed. London 1861.

Smith, Ginnie: Prescribing the Rules of Health: Self-Help and Advice in the Late Eighteenth Century. In: Porter, Roy (ed.): Patients and Practitioners: Lay Perceptions of Medicine in Pre-Industrial Society. Cambridge 1985, pp. 249–282.

South, John F.: Household Surgery: Or, Hints on Emergencies. 4th ed. London 1852.

Stearns, Carol Zisowitz; Stearns, Peter N.: Anger: The Struggle for Emotional Control in America's History. Chicago; London 1986.

Stine, Jennifer K.: Opening Closets: The Discovery of Household Medicine in Early Modern England. Unpublished PhD thesis, Stanford University 1996.

Stobart, Anne: The Making of Domestic Medicine: Gender, Self-Help and Therapeutic Determinism in Household Healthcare in South-West England in the Late Seventeenth Century. Unpublished PhD thesis, University of Middlesex 2008.

Thomson, Spencer: A Dictionary of Domestic Medicine and Household Surgery. 24th ed. revised by J. C. Steele, assisted by the author. London [1882?].

Ueyama, Takahiro: Health in the Marketplace. Professionalism, Therapeutic Desires, and Medical Commodification in Late-Victorian London. Palo Alto, CA 2010.

Walsh, J. H.: Domestic Medicine and Surgery. New revised ed. London 1875.

Medical Pluralism in Britain 1850–1930

Phillip A. Nicholls

Introduction

The title of the paper suggests a daunting array of therapies, each with its own story to tell, and each with its own peculiar evolutionary trajectory. Any attempt to cover all of this ground would be exhausting, both for the author of this paper and, I suspect, for my readers too. Hence, rather than trying to summarise and describe the history of each individual therapy I shall attempt to uncover – or, perhaps more modestly, suggest – from a sociological perspective, some features which they have in common, and to propose and account for an overall pattern in the development of 'fringe medicine' during the period under consideration here. To do so effectively, however, I will need to plead for a little licence in trespassing, to some extent, beyond the time frame specified in the title.

Regular and Irregular Medicine

The first, and I suspect least contentious point to make, is that the binary opposition of 'regular' and 'irregular' medicine necessarily implies the notion of 'rejected knowledge'. An influential view here is that the boundary between accepted and rejected knowledge is neutrally and objectively drawn by the disinterested investigation of the knowledge claim or claims in question – for example, through the application of the scientific method. However, as philosophers and sociologists of science have pointed out, from the pioneering work of Thomas Kuhn[1] onwards, this account is historically and empirically naive as it fails to recognise that the acceptance or rejection of knowledge claims is a social process, undertaken by social actors, in particular social contexts, who may well have particular interests to pursue and defend (for example, theoretical paradigms around which professional reputations, incomes, research budgets, careers, and political influence have been built).

This process is visible, of course, in the professionalisation of medicine. It is a barely contestable point – to take the most obvious example – that the Medical Act of 1858 was a product of vigorously pursued occupational interests, and that its intended effect was to strengthen doctors' position in the market for medical care and employment by creating an identifiable fringe of practitioners who, lacking the educational qualifications required for registration, had to be regarded with scepticism by state and public alike – as 'healers'

---

1 Kuhn (1962).

whose 'knowledge' was suspect, and whose therapeutic approach and remedies were either worthless or dangerous. Here, then, occupational interests
were triumphant in creating a therapeutic 'other' or 'outsider'. Whether practitioners were unqualified, or whether they were eligible for medical registration but chose to pursue a mode of practice not embodied in the standard
curriculum of the medical schools, the political interests of the profession had
successfully demarcated acceptable from unacceptable kinds of healing knowledge and practice.

This point, though an obvious and powerful one to make, is sometimes at
risk of closing off further historical research and debate. Such an outcome
would be unfortunate, as there is much, much more which needs to be investigated in terms of the social history of alternative medicine, and in terms of
the particular histories of the individual therapies which comprise the field itself. What I want to propose here, however, is that these individual histories
nevertheless seem to share certain features which allow a general historical
pattern of development to be discerned.

This development, I suggest, begins with a situation where irregular medicine is, first, a pastiche of regular practice to one where, by the middle decades
of the nineteenth century, it is to be understood not only as a rejection of orthodox medicine but also as an expression of political dissent in a rapidly in-
dustrialising society. The third phase of development is one of virtual eclipse
and exhaustion. This final period is characteristic of the early decades of the
twentieth century.

In a sense, the historical trajectory proposed here can be understood, at
the most general level, as akin to a dialectical movement: the relatively undifferentiated totality of therapeutic practice in the eighteenth and early nineteenth century moves, first, to division and contestation among practitioners
and then, eventually, to a reconstituted homogeneity. It is this overall trend
which I want to explore in more detail, and which I shall try to account for, in
what remains of the paper.

The pattern of development suggested above, incidentally and intriguingly, seems to repeat itself in the second half of the twentieth century, with
the unrivalled prestige and dominance of regular medicine first coming under
critique and attack around the 1970s, both from political radicals like Illich[2]
(whose gospel of self-help where health was concerned bears some remarkable similarities to the message preached by many advocates of irregular practice in the nineteenth century), and from a reinvigorated field of alternative,
'holistic' therapy which pointed, first and foremost, to the iatrogenic consequences of industrial, professionalised medicine. This period of contestation
has, more recently, been followed by one of gradual rapprochement and incorporation, where previously stigmatised 'alternative' therapies have increasingly become a 'complementary' aspect of publicly funded health care.

2   Illich (1977).

It would be fascinating to explore in more detail just how far the similarities between the developmental cycle of relations between regular and irregular medicine in the nineteenth and twentieth centuries might be pressed, but that is perhaps a task for a future paper. It is necessary here, however, to turn to the first claim made about the nature of the dialectical trajectory proposed above – that in the eighteenth and early nineteenth centuries therapeutic practice represented a relatively undifferentiated totality in so far as irregular healers, in the main, operated in the medical market with much the same kinds of commercial strategies and remedies as those entitled to claim the title 'doctor'.

This particular thesis has been argued extensively by Roy Porter.[3] He suggests that, particularly for the eighteenth century, it is dangerous to write about the delivery and consumption of health care from the perspective of qualified practice. To do so, he contends, risks dividing the field into those who had been formally trained and held a licence to practise and 'the rest' – the 'reputable' irregulars, like most bone-setters, or the founder of Methodism, John Wesley (see, for example, his widely read 'Primitive Physick', first published in 1747)[4], and then the quacks, the fraudsters and the confidence tricksters. Not merely does this strategy beg important questions – firstly, about competence (for many 'quacks' were competent in their own right and many who held licences patently were not) and, secondly, about the sincerity of intentions (for neither can it be assumed that all 'quacks' were insincere) – it also obscures the impact of the growth of the new consumer society on the way in which medical services were provided. All practitioners, qualified or not, were subject to the same kinds of economic exigencies in terms of their employment, and all used the same kinds of strategies – and even remedies – to survive.

Instead, Porter suggests, it is better to see the eighteenth century medical milieu as a totality distinguished by four principal characteristics: low therapeutic efficacy, a high degree of pluralism, a high degree of consumer choice and lay participation, and the rise of a new market based medical consumerism.

Illness was an ever-present reality for all classes in eighteenth century Britain. The sick, however, in terms of relief and cure, could really find little difference between the medication prescribed by physicians and mixed by apothecaries and the patented and proprietary medicines peddled by quacks or available at the shop counter. The same principal ingredients – such as opium, antimony, mercury and powerful purgative agents – tended to characterise both.

This lack of therapeutic efficacy simply encouraged medical pluralism to flourish. The free market – even in London, where the writ of the Royal College of Physicians (RCP) supposedly imposed restrictions on practice – gave rise to a new class of medical entrepreneurs. Among the more socially and

3   Amongst his many relevant publications in this area see Porter (1988; 1989) and also
     Porter/Porter (1989).
4   Wesley (1747).

economically successful of these were practitioners such as Joshua 'spot' Ward (famous for his 'drop' and his attractively coloured pills, which contained antimony and arsenic as their main ingredients), the oculist John 'the Chevalier' Taylor, Sally Mapp – a bone-setter who was consulted even by the President of the RCP – and James Graham, noted for the risqué lectures which he delivered in conjunction with the deliberately concupiscent spectacles provided in his 'Temple of Health'. This new entrepreneurial spirit was often matched by many among the qualified: William Hunter, for example – who established a private anatomy school – is representative of such market orientated initiatives.

Since the Crown itself could provide licenses to practise to whomsoever it chose, and since the government could derive considerable revenue from applications by empirics to patent any particular nostrum, it was clear that 'medical pluralism' had official sanction. An extensive range of healers, specialising in particular forms of practice or promoting certain kinds of remedies, from the top physicians of the Royal Court down to the humblest bone-setter or tooth drawer, were able to work freely and also, especially where brand leading patented or proprietary remedies, such as Dr James's Powders were purveyed, lucratively. The chance for fame and economic reward, whether qualified or not, lay in the deft exploitation of the medical market place and in self-promotion. In its most flamboyant form, this manifested itself via the staging of exhibitions, events, entertainments and spectacles. Improved methods of communication and transportation also played their role in the endeavour to win market advantage: healers could celebrate themselves and their remedies in newspapers and journals and via hand bills and pamphlets distributed or displayed in coffee houses or other public spaces; postal services enhanced the ability to distribute products; and the shop counters of the flourishing retail sector could display nostrums cleverly branded to appeal to fashionable society.

Thus it is hard to see, for the eighteenth century, any strict divide between mere 'commercial' and 'professional' practice. Both were shaped by the same economic interests, and both were in the same subordinate position in relation to their clients – a situation which Jewson[5] has famously conceptualised as a system of patronage where the particular forms of therapeutic approach advocated by different healers multiplied as each jostled for market advantage and distinctiveness[6].

In this sense the period is quite distinctive from that which followed. In the nineteenth century it was increasingly seen as imperative to draw a line between 'regular' and 'irregular' practice as a way of preventing the contamination of the former by the latter, and as a way of legitimating the regular profession's new claims on the state for occupational privilege and protection. At the same time the growth of hospital based medicine began significantly to transfer power from patients to doctors: in turn, this helped the profession to

5   Jewson (1974).
6   Jewson (1976); Nicolson (1988).

organise and educate itself around a more uniform and codified body of therapeutic knowledge.

There is one other important regard in which irregular practice in the two
centuries differs: the eighteenth century empiric was very firmly working in
the new commercial spirit of the age, and essentially with the same kinds of
remedies, as the respectably qualified physician or surgeon-apothecary. The
forging of therapeutic links with politics or religion was avoided because it was
commercially dangerous. His nineteenth century successor was, however, a
very different (and, one cannot help suspecting, rather less appealing) character, defined not only by a rejection of medical orthodoxy and the celebration
of more 'natural' ways of healing but also, not uncommonly, by an opposi-
tional politics and a dissenting religion.

Porter summarises the overall situation as follows:

> Eighteenth century quackery colluded, rather than collided, with regular medicine. It did
> not set itself up as the champion of alternative systems of healing, replete with radical
> medical ontologies and distinctive therapies. Rather, market-place medicine essentially
> shared or pirated the ideas and pillaged the practices of the establishment, seeking to
> render its medicines more accessible, sometimes cheaper, and more palatable to the buy-
> ers (and more profitable to the purveyors) by economies of scale and perfection of the art
> of selling.[7]

Homoeopathy

The most serious challenge to the regular profession in the nineteenth century,
however, came from practitioners who certainly did see themselves as the
champions of a genuinely alternative system of medicine – the homoeopaths
– who, in stark contrast to those doctors they now described as 'allopaths',
advocated the use of symptomatically 'similar' rather than opposing remedies,
working with the healing processes of the body rather than instead of or
against them, and the use of 'infinitesimal' rather than toxic doses of remedies.

The story behind this headline, though, is both more subtle and more
complex than might first appear to be the case.[8] It had not, after all, been the
first intention of the early homoeopathic doctors in Britain to declare therapeutic warfare. Dr Frederick Foster Hervey Quin (1798–1878) – who was in
large measure responsible for the construction of the early institutional apparatus of homoeopathy in Britain – was not a radical by temperament or incli-
nation. On the contrary, he was cultured and popular within aristocratic circles; he preferred to see homoeopathy as a particularly useful therapeutic approach, but one which might, on occasion, need support from more orthodox
interventions; and he was most concerned to preserve good relations with the
regular profession by jealously guarding the professional integrity of homoeopathy and its practitioners. It was no surprise, then, to find that Quin simply

7 Porter (1988), p. 14.
8 Nicholls (1988).

reproduced the typical organisational structures of regular medicine in giving institutional identity to homoeopathy: he founded the British Homoeopathic Society (BHS), together with its associated journal, the *British Journal of Homoeopathy*, in 1844, and worked tirelessly with the British Homoeopathic Association to raise funds for the foundation of the London Homoeopathic Hospital, which opened in 1850.

Quin's desire for good professional relations with his allopathic colleagues, however, was sabotaged by the growing campaign for medical reform led by figures like Thomas Wakley (1795–1862), the radical editor of *The Lancet*. Wakely had long been concerned to raise the incomes, status and educational standards of the ordinary general practitioner, and of engaging the state in securing a privileged position for regular, licensed practitioners in terms of private practice and public employment. This was eventually realised, of course, in the form of the Medical Act of 1858. Inevitably, however, as part of this process, Wakley had waged a ferocious war against what he regarded as 'quackery': after all, if the regular profession was not confident enough in itself to distinguish between competent and dangerous practice, why should the state listen to its pleas for occupational protection? Equally inevitably, homoeopathy fell very squarely among the range of therapies from which a gullible public needed safeguarding so far as Wakley and his supporters were concerned.

What followed was a systematic campaign of vilification of those doctors who were prepared to call themselves homoeopaths, and their exclusion from regular medical societies, from consultations with orthodox practitioners, and their employment in hospitals other than those which were homoeopathic. This process of ostracism was begun at the nineteenth annual meeting of the Provincial Medical and Surgical Association (later the British Medical Association) in 1851. In effect, the professionalising strategies of regular practitioners had solidified a therapeutic divide between homoeopaths and other doctors which Quin and his early colleagues had never intended: the result was a division which was as much a consequence of ostracism as it was its cause.[9]

Quin and his followers, however, while being progressively cast as therapeutic pariahs by the orthodox profession, were also subject to attack by some homoeopaths themselves. It is this group of practitioners who first begin to reveal what I will argue to be some of the distinguishing characteristics of unorthodox medicine in general in the middle decades of the nineteenth century – political and social radicalism coupled with therapeutic dissent. The career of John Epps (1805–1869) nicely illustrates the point in question.

Epps was a political libertarian, a strong democrat, a deeply religious nonconformist, and was involved in many popular movements for social reform.[10] Before converting to homoeopathy, he had been an advocate of phrenology. Epps was a supporter of the anti-slavery movement, of the anti-Corn

9   Nicholls (2001).
10 Much of the text on Epps and Quin first appeared in Nicholls (2010), pp. 286–287.

Law League, of moderate Chartism, and was an enthusiastic writer and speaker who regularly addressed working men's associations throughout the country. For Epps, it was at least as important to address a self-helping, self-improving wider public on these matters as it was to speak to professional or other more refined audiences.

These political orientations and sympathies were almost bound to clash with someone of Quin's temperament and affiliations. Quin's view of the relationship between homoeopathy and its public (where the 'knowledgeable expert' would act in 'the best interests' of an untutored and dependent clientele) mirrored the reforming orientation of the Whig aristocracy (among whom he had many friends): social reform was to be pursued, but only if it was managed by the governing class for the people, who needed a benevolent and enlightened elite to help them.

John Epps, however, had a very different perspective. His views were much more obviously populist, anti-elitist and democratic. For Epps, reform needed to take account of the views of those affected by the reforms themselves. Moreover, especially where homoeopathy was concerned, it seemed clear enough that the 'raw materials of illness', and therefore of remedy selection, were not wrapped in esoteric knowledge, but were available to all as the symptomatic expression of disease. In managing their health, just as in managing other aspects of their lives, people could, armed with the appropriate knowledge, improve and help themselves without the interference of social, intellectual or political 'superiors'[11] (it is easy to see, then, why homoeopaths of Epps' persuasion produced and published so many domestic guides to homoeopathic principles and practice).

These contrasting political orientations emerged as soon as Quin began his work on building the institutional apparatus of homoeopathy. Epps made it very clear that he felt that the constitution of the BHS as proposed by its President gave Quin far too much power. Epps withdrew from Quin's circle and then joined with more like-minded others, such as Paul Curie (1799–1853) and lay supporters like Mr Sampson, Mr Heurtley and Mr Leaf – to form the English Homoeopathic Association (EHA) in 1845. Membership of the Association reflected the more democratic and populist principles favoured by Epps and others: membership was open to both medical and lay supporters, whose main aim would be to promote knowledge about and use of homoeopathy among the general public. Pointedly, its first publication ('Homoeopathy: Its Principle, Theory and Practice')[12] was written by a layperson – the banker and journalist Marmaduke Sampson. Quin would never have tolerated this collusion of the professional and popular worlds on medical matters.

The discussion of this second phase of the developmental cycle in the relations between regular and irregular medicine had, almost inevitably, to begin with homoeopathy, as it was one of the most powerful of the therapeutic threats to allopathic hegemony during the middle decades of the nineteenth

11 These points are also made by Rankin (1988).
12 Sampson (1845).

century. Yet to begin with a discussion of homoeopathy is also potentially mis-
leading for the simple reason that the 'respectable' wing of the movement
founded and led by Quin left by far the more enduring institutional legacy –
not least because of the parliamentary protection which homoeopathy's aristocratic and royal supporters were prepared to provide. The kind of 'populist'
homoeopathy preferred by Epps – which emphasised its wholesomeness, its
spiritual properties and its ability to help the layperson treat themselves – res-
onated among the workers of the northern mill towns, such as Rochdale in
Lancashire[13], where evangelical religious dissent, especially Methodism, was
strong, but was certainly less appealing to the majority of homoeopathy's
more socially privileged supporters.

Nevertheless, the dissenting voices raised by Epps and the EHA against
Quin's presidency expressed the themes which would tend to characterise the
particular non-conformities of many of the followers of other irregular therapeutic approaches during this period, such as hydrotherapy, botanical medicine, mesmerism and spiritualism. It is true enough that the newly emerging
entrepreneurial and industrial bourgeoisie of the period were generally sympathetic to the claims of irregular practitioners, simply because they supported
free trade, and disliked as a matter of principle the monopolistic aspirations of
the regular medical profession, but we need to look a little deeper than this
unsurprising fact if we are to uncover the particular appeal of irregular practice to those groups in society dissenting in different ways from the prevailing
social order.

Supporters of irregular practice were often also, as has been seen, members of evangelical non-conformist religious groups and/or were part of political movements, such as Chartism, or were supporters of the co-operative socialism of Robert Owen (1771–1858). Such groups were either primarily re-
sentful of the overweening power of the established Church, or were keen to
limit the power of the state over the individual through the defence of a radical individualism or via the extension in various ways of democratic rights.
The key aspirations in each case revolve around the ideas of 'self-help', 'personal autonomy' and – crucially – 'self-government'. Quite simply, the most
popular of the irregular therapies in the nineteenth century offered ordinary
citizens the chance to govern themselves in the matter of health in the same
way as they wished to govern themselves in the matters of religion, politics or
work. After all, running through all of the major therapeutic rivals of orthodox
medicine in the period were the themes of naturalism and transparency – the
therapies were derived from nature, were 'wholesome' (and so perhaps had
Divine endorsement) and were 'transparent' in the sense that they could be
understood and practised by the layperson without the supervision of any professional elite. In short, the reason why many members of religiously and politically dissenting groups in the nineteenth century were often also supporters

13   Pickstone (1982), see especially pp. 177–183.

of the major irregular therapies of the period was, I would argue, that both kinds of affiliation were an expression of the same desire for self-government.

Hydropathy

Hydropathy, which emerged in Britain in the 1840s, provides a further illustration of this tendency. The system first came to the country's serious attention via the work of Captain Richard T. Claridge, who had travelled from Rome in 1841 to seek the help of hydropathy's founder, Vincent Priessnitz (1799–1851), for relief from chronic headache and rheumatism.[14] Claridge's book, 'Hydropathy; or, the Cold Water Cure, as Practised by Vincent Priessnitz, at Graefenberg, Silesia, Austria'[15], left his readers in no doubt of his belief in the efficacy of this new form of treatment. His work found an early and eager readership, reaching a third edition in the first year of its publication.

Like homoeopathy, hydropathy came to be patronised in Britain by many leading social figures (for example, Lord Tennyson, Charles Darwin, Thomas Carlyle and Florence Nightingale)[16], as well as by members of the fashion conscious aristocracy. Hydropathy's clientele, however, again like homoeopathy, was not confined to these groupings. By 1891, Britain had sixty-three major hydropathic centres, with particular concentrations around the rural towns of Malvern, Ilkely and Matlock, but there were many smaller establishments which attracted the 'respectable' working classes.[17]

Hydropathy shared other characteristics, too, with homoeopathy: indeed, many hydropaths, like those centred on Malvern, as well as Doctors William Mcleod and William Forbes Laurie, were keen advocates and practitioners of both systems.[18] Firstly, both therapies were practised by qualified doctors as well as by lay persons. As far as the regular profession was concerned, both systems were heresies, and both received the usual literary lashings from medical journals such as *The Lancet*, although the attacks on hydropathy were less severe, and less prolonged, on the whole, than they were on homoeopathy. After all, as Price points out[19], most educated physicians were aware of the tradition of water based treatments in conventional practice from the eighteenth century onwards. In both cases, too, the issues of medical respectability and acceptability tended to create similar tensions between regularly qualified hydropaths and those who practised the system without a medical licence.

Secondly, homoeopathy and hydropathy both celebrated the healing power of Nature, criticised the regular profession's damaging addiction to heroic drugging, bleeding and blistering, and aimed to assist the natural healing

14   Price (1981), p. 272.
15   Claridge (1842).
16   Price (1981), pp. 277, 280.
17   Rees (1988), p. 28.
18   Brown (1987), p. 227.
19   Price (1981), p. 271.

processes of the human body in a holistic way. Hydropathy, as developed by Priessnitz, however, proceeded to do so in a manner quite distinct to that of homoeopathy: to opt for hydropathic treatment required a degree of physical courage and moral determination quite unlike anything experienced by a patient of a homoeopath.

At the core of Priessnitz's system is the familiar idea that illness is to be understood as a product of foreign matter introduced into the human organism; that acute disease should be seen as the body's attempt to rid itself of peccant material; and that only water is able to remove this morbid matter from the human system. Drugging and bleeding only serve to push disease 'inwards' and this results in chronic disease. Hydropathic treatment is the only way of tackling this morbidity by forcing an acute crisis (manifested, for example, in an eruption of boils) in which water treatments (baths, wet blankets, douches and the consumption of heroic quantities of cold water) can help to combat and 'carry off' the diseased material. In addition – and these were the great prophylactic regimes which gave the system therapeutic integrity – water treatments were to be conjoined with fresh air, exercise, a good diet and a temperate life style. In this way, good health could be both regained and retained.

As reformulated in Britain by doctors such as James Wilson (d. 1867) and James Gully (1808–1883), and by lay practitioners such as John Smedley (1803–1876)[20], hydropathy lost some of Priessnitz's hypothermic zeal. The account of the disease process also came to focus more on depleted levels of energy than the intrusion of morbid material – but in the basic emphasis on the cycle of water based therapeutic interventions, the idea of 'crisis', and the need for clean living, exercise, temperance, a good diet and moral circumspection, the system remained, in essentials, much the same.

There were themes, then, embedded within hydropathic philosophy – a simple and transparent account of disease, and of its treatment and prevention, which could be understood and practised by non-professionals; the ideas of naturalism and purity; and the prophylactic effects of temperance and discipline – that were readily attractive to the religious rebel, as well as to the self-made entrepreneur and the self-improving artisan and worker. John Smedley provides a good example of both the first and second types.

Smedley had succeeded in returning to profitability a failing family spinning and hosiery business in Matlock and, having experienced successful hydropathic treatment in Harrogate in 1851 for a long-standing nervous ailment, opened a free hospital based on the new treatment for his workers. In 1853, he took over an eleven bedroomed hydropathic establishment in Matlock. By 1869 Smedley had seen this business grow to 172 bedrooms which catered for some 2,000 patients per year. Concurrently, Smedley had forsaken Anglicanism and became a leading promoter of, and lay preacher for, the United Free Methodist Church. For Smedley, then, hydropathy, with its naturalistic ap-

---

20   Gully (1846); Wilson (1857); Smedley (1858).

proach, its endorsement of temperance and moral discipline, and with the accessibility of its theory and practice to the untutored layperson, provided the perfect therapeutic benediction for both his commercial success and his religious dissent. Not surprisingly, Smedley was not the only lay hydropath to have found the system a natural accompaniment to their religious non-conformity or interest in temperance: Brown, for example, mentions among others Archibald Hunter, Spencer T. Hall, Samuel Kenworthy, Edward Johnson, Ralph Grindrod and Abraham Courtney.[21]

Smedley's 'Practical Hydropathy' – which eventually ran to fifteen editions, and had alone sold some 85,000 copies by 1872 – is a measure in itself of the popularity of the system, and also of its attractiveness to such as self-improving artisans, and members of the 'respectable operative classes'[22], who could afford to come to the many smaller hydropathic establishments in Matlock and elsewhere. The working man could govern himself, his life and his family in matters of health through the deployment of hydropathic principles, without dependence on obscure knowledge which needed to be mediated by professionals, in the same way that he might seek to take better control of his life-chances in the worlds of work, politics and religion.

If it was easy enough for the self-improving working class and religious dissenters to find a political ally in hydropathy, then the arrival in Britain of another therapeutic movement – medical botany – had perhaps even greater appeal. Indeed, the ideas of self-help and self-governance, of a demystified medicine which could be of and for the people, were explicitly inscribed within the principles of the system itself, and were cogently articulated by its leading figures.

Herbalism

Herbalism had a long tradition as folk medicine in Britain, and the memory of its domestic use was still within the reach of the emerging working class in the early industrial centres of the nineteenth century. This certainly helped to lay a foundation for the enthusiastic response which the arrival of medical botany elicited, especially amongst workers in the more remote, but pioneering manufacturing centres in the north of England. Based on Thomsonian medicine which had been flourishing in America – where the principle of self-help had long assumed the status of a virtuous necessity to early pioneers and settlers – medical botany owed its early promotion to the efforts of Dr Albert Isaiah Coffin (1790/91–1866)[23], who came to England in 1838 (the unfortunate implications of his name were not, of course, lost on those who sought to protect the medical profession and the public from so-called 'quackery'). Coffin, though, if the most renowned of medical botany's founding figures, was not

21   Brown (1987), pp. 224, 226.
22   Rees (1988), p. 34.
23   See his exposition of the system in Coffin (1846).

the first to have practised Thomsonian medicine in Britain: Samuel Westcott Tilke, a baker, and Dr Whitelaw of East Lothian in Scotland, as well as the brothers George and John Stevens in Bristol, had been practising similar system prior to 1838.[24] Neither did Coffinism immediately and entirely displace the more traditional herbal practitioners: rather, the two kinds of practitioners co-existed, and actual practice often tended to overlap.[25]

Coffinism, however, as practised in its pure form (and Coffin had a tendency to split with any medical botanist who deviated from the principles he had articulated in his 'Botanic Guide'), had a perfectly distinctive theory of disease and of how it should be treated. His approach had, on the one hand, apparently little time for the tailored prescriptions of the traditional herbalist (or for those of homoeopaths or hydropaths for that matter) and, on the other, a disdain for the obscurantism and violent drugging fashionable among regular doctors. Ironically, however, what it put in their place was a monocausal theory of disease and a standardised system of treatment which, like hydropathy, could require some degree of physical courage to complete. For Coffin, the basis of disease was loss of heat, and the objective of treatment was to restore warmth to the human system by the use of herbal remedies (most often, Lobelia – an emetic – and Cayenne Pepper), steam baths (it was, after all, the age of steam), and warming teas.

Coffinism, then, was principally characterised by its violent attacks on the regular profession, by its claim to embrace Nature and her healing properties and processes in its therapeutic approach, by its distrust of professionalism, and by its advocacy of a demystified medicine which would 'enable the millions [in Britain] to prescribe for themselves'.[26] Coffin himself was, of course, a populist. He propagated his system via skilfully composed and convincing – to the common person at least – public lectures, which were delivered with missionary zeal. Like Thomson in America, he aimed to establish local botanical societies: members were required to purchase copies of his 'Botanic Guide', and to pay a fee of six shillings. Society members were expected to visit and prescribe for the sick, and to report back to society meetings on interesting cases and successful treatments. However, while a number of such societies were established in Yorkshire and Lancashire, Coffin also seems, again like Thomson, to have used agents to prescribe and sell his medicines (provided the agents had satisfied Coffin of their proficiency in, and strict adherence to, his system).

Coffinism was certainly popular: in the 1850s, the *Medical Times* estimated that there were about 6,000 irregular practitioners in Britain, and that medical botanists represented a large proportion of this number.[27] Coffin himself claimed that, by 1864, 40,000 copies of his book had been sold, and that his

24   Brown (1982), p. 408; Miley/Pickstone (1988), p. 145.
25   Brown (1982), p. 417.
26   Brown (1982), p. 410.
27   Brown (1982), p. 412.

Botanical Journal, which appeared fortnightly, had a circulation of 10,000[28] –
but these figures should be treated with some caution: there is no independent
verification of the data, and Coffin was, of course, well-schooled in the art of
self-promotion.

For our purposes, however, it is crucial to identify the social groups who
formed a special allegiance to botanical medicine, and to inquire about their
particular political and religious sympathies. Coffin himself had first made for
London when he arrived in England; he then moved to Hull, and by 1844 had
established himself in Manchester. There he tutored John Skelton in botanical
practice; significantly, Skelton had signed the People's Charter in 1838 and
had also been a leading Chartist in the metropolis. The two were to work in
close partnership (for a while at least, before an acrimonious separation) and
toured many northern and midland towns together in order to promote the
gospel of 'the people's medicine' (visiting places such as Rotherham, Black-
burn, Oldham, Wakefield, Barnsley, Stockport, Birmingham, Manchester,
Derby, Nottingham and Leicester).[29] By the 1850s, Skelton had established
his own practice, first in Leeds and then in Manchester.

The main strength, then, of the botanic movement, and the majority of its
followers, seems to have been concentrated in the north of the country. This
was probably no accident, for in England the early development of industry
had taken place in the north-west of the country, a region then far removed, of
course, from the metropolis, and a region in which the power of traditional
social and religious elites was correspondingly weaker. Dissent – in the form
of Wesleyan Methodism and emerging demands for political reform – had already established itself in such areas. Pickstone, who makes this point[30], then
goes on to elaborate the particular political and religious proclivities (noted
also, incidentally, by Brown, Harrison and Miley)[31] of many of botanical
medicine's strongest adherents:

> [...] by the 1840s in the industrial areas of Britain there were large numbers of more or
> less literate artisans, shopkeepers and factory workers who, schooled in the organisations
> of Dissent, were liberal-radical or radical in politics, democratic in temper, thirsty for sci-
> ence and deeply interested in self-improvement – as a religious duty, as a means of self
> advancement, or as a contribution to the advancement of their class. There is a similarity
> of temper extending from those whose major interest was Chartism, through those whose
> major public commitment was religious, to those radical-liberals who for various reasons
> identified themselves with artisans and small manufacturers.[32]

Coffinism, then, was a natural ally of religious dissenters: Coffin, after all,
propagated his system with the same missionary zeal employed by Wesleyan
Methodists. Often the bulk of his audiences and many of his followers were
dissenters, and botanical societies frequently met in Wesleyan or Primitive

28   Miley/Pickstone (1988), p. 150.
29   Harrison (1987), p. 200.
30   Pickstone (1976/77), p. 88.
31   Brown (1982); Harrison (1987); Miley/Pickstone (1988).
32   Pickstone (1976/77), pp. 89–90.

Methodist Chapels – or, significantly, in Halls devoted to the temperance movement, in which Coffinism easily found a further ally.[33] It was also the friend, on the political side, of those, like Chartists and Owenite Socialists, who were interested in the extension of democratic rights. Botanical medicine, then, was an obvious ally of both, since it was simply a further extension – into the field of health – of the desire for self-determination, improvement and governance which had underpinned and motivated other forms of political, religious and social dissent.

Mesmerism and Spiritualism

The same constellation of interests came to be seen among many of the supporters and practitioners of mesmerism and spiritualism. 'Animal Magnetism' had first flourished in France in the 1770s and 1780s, and had arisen from Anton Mesmer's (1734–1815) conviction that he had discovered an invisible force or fluid that was omnipresent in all things, both animate and inanimate, in the universe. For human beings, this meant that illness could be explained as a disruption of the natural ebb and flow of this fluid through the body. Further, Mesmer noted that some people could apparently affect and re-balance this flow by passing their hands in rhythmic patterns over a patient's body, and thus restore health.

Mesmerism became extremely popular in Britain from 1837 onwards.[34] It had first been introduced by a formidable medical figure, Dr John Elliotson (1791–1868), Professor of Medicine at the University of London. From that point onwards, Elliotson led a small group of medical mesmerists, who flourished in the 1840s and during the first years of the following decade. Elliotson claimed that mesmerism was especially useful in treating patients with neurological disorders – and that it had particular potential as an anaesthetic during surgery.[35]

Elliotson, however, paid for his enthusiasm with professional dishonour. He was forced to resign his professorship at the university, and his mesmeric investigations and demonstrations there were judged to have brought the College into disrepute. This was not surprising in the climate of the times, for the regular profession reacted as violently to the therapeutic claims of mesmerism as it had to other kinds of irregular practice. Medical men disliked the fact that Mesmer's ideas challenged prevailing conceptions of disease and its treatment; they objected to the fact that mesmerism undermined the idea of healing as a reserve of the professionally trained and qualified (since it could be practised by anyone); and they railed against its impact on medical incomes as potential patients began to seek out or practise mesmeric healing. Furthermore, mesmerism was felt to be additionally dishonourable and unprofes-

33   Miley/Pickstone (1988), p. 148.
34   Parssinen (1979), p. 106.
35   Parssinen (1979), pp. 106–107.

sional because it seemed to have links with ancient magical/religious forms of healing 'by touch'; because it seemed to give the practitioner dangerous power over clients rendered defenceless by mesmeric trance; and because, as Parssinen points out, by the 1830s and 1840s:

> Self-proclaimed 'professors' of the subject swarmed throughout the kingdom, demonstrating their subjects' clairvoyant powers through 'experiments' in which the entranced subjects would read from a book or paper while blindfolded.[36]

For medical men such displays, where typically medical mesmerism would also be offered and promoted to individual members of the audience on a private basis, seemed to be:

> [...] a reincarnation of the seventeenth and eighteenth-century tradition of medical mountebanks, who performed a short entertainment before hawking their patent medicines at fairs and carnivals. It was bad enough that the public equated medical men with tradesmen; would they now equate them with showmen as well?[37]

Elliotson, then, and his fellow medical enthusiasts, were definitely in the minority: most mesmerists were not professionally qualified. This, of course, for our purposes, is the nub of the issue: as a system with therapeutic applications, mesmerism was open, democratic, transferable and transparent. In so far as it was a gift which some people had, or could hone and perfect, it was not, and could not be, the preserve of any closed professional elite. Therein lay its attraction to political radicals and reformers. A very significant minority of Owenites and Chartists, as Harrison points out[38], were thus, predictably enough, also supporters and practitioners of mesmerism.

Where mesmerism had led, spiritualism followed. The two systems were often practised together, and they both appealed to the same politically conscious groupings, and for the same reasons. In 1854, aged 83, Robert Owen himself had decided to follow a route already taken by many of his sympathisers and followers, and became a convert to spiritualism.[39]

In one sense, the attraction of Owenites and Chartists to spiritualism ran counter to what might have been expected, given the secular orientation of both movements, and in particular in view of the hostile attitude of Owen and his followers to religion and the established church. To be sure, spiritualism was anti-professional, open and democratic in its ethos, and represented a way of putting within the control of ordinary people answers to important life issues without the mediation of self-interested experts or other elites – and these themes, of course, chimed well with the aspirations of many radicals. But it needs also to be remembered that by the end of the 1840s the momentum had begun to drain away from both Chartism and Owenite socialism, and spiritualism seems to have presented itself, as Barrow suggests[40], as a form of reas-

36   Parssinen (1979), p. 113.
37   Parssinen (1979), p. 113.
38   Harrison (1987), p. 198.
39   Harrison (1987), pp. 198–199; Barrow (1982), p. 226.
40   Barrow (1982), pp. 232–233.

surance that all had not been in vain – that there was something beyond death which meant that a life spent in the service of self-improvement would in some way live on.

Spiritualism was unique in a number of ways when compared to other irregular forms of healing. Firstly, it elicited a very distinctive response from regular medical men and from other professional scientists – not least because some very distinguished scientific figures, such as Alfred Russell Wallace, were converts and advocates – but also because of the way in which the sceptics organised a systematic investigation of mediums and of the phenomena which they produced during séances. Not surprisingly, much of this investigative work employed magicians and conjurors, who were asked to reproduce the effects associated with spiritualist practice, and thereby expose the assumed fraud. This is a distinctive and fascinating story, well told by Palfreman[41], but it is not one, however, that it would be quite appropriate to explore further here. Secondly, spiritualism offered special opportunities to women (and it was certainly the case that most spiritualist healers were women)[42] to advance themselves as professional healers, a role which the regular medical world, of course, denied them. Here, the very qualities ascribed to women which confined them to subordinate roles in both the public and private spheres – passivity and receptivity – were exactly the traits which made for special expertise and deftness in the role of medium.

Spiritualism arrived in Britain from America in 1852, when the first professional medium, Mrs Hayden, was introduced by Mr Stone.[43] By 1853, 'table-turning', as it came to be called, had become almost a national pastime.[44] Public fascination with the phenomena was to peak again in the 1870s and 1880s: by then, total membership of those loose organisations which made up plebeian spiritualism was over 10,000.[45]

Spiritualism was another of those irregular houses of healing which welcomed all-comers. It was a therapeutic endeavour which, like others, belonged to the people rather than to any profession. All that was needed was the recognition and cultivation of the special powers required for successful practice, and anyone, of course, might be so blessed. Mediumistic healing, however, was usually regarded as the highest gift of all, and was closely associated with mesmeric theory. As Owen explains:

> When a mesmerised practitioner offered a complete diagnosis based on her ability to 'see' into the body of a patient, or a healer explained that she was exchanging her positive energy for another's depleted vitality, each assumed that the process was facilitated by an extension of magnetic or electro-biological fluid.[46]

41   Palfreman (1979).
42   Owen (1989), pp. 112–113.
43   Palfreman (1979), p. 203.
44   Palfreman (1979), p. 204.
45   Barrow (1982), p. 232.
46   Owen (1989), p. 109.

In short, the effective healer used the spirit world for guidance in diagnosis and treatment (or sometimes simply to act as a channel for a healing spirit), and mesmeric energy as the therapeutic intervention.

Social class also emerges as a factor in understanding spiritualist practice. Working class women tended to operate as healers in the public domain for money; middle class women, on the other hand, tended to practise in the domestic sphere among friends and family – a situation where any consideration of a fee would, of course, be inappropriate. Whatever their social origins, however, mediumistic healers presented their gift as a naturalistic phenomenon and their craft as holistic: drugging and doctors, under this regime, became irrelevant and dangerous. It was democratic medicine, open to all as healer or client. It was also, as celebrated by famous healers such as Chandos Leigh Hunt, a practice which should ideally be conjoined with rigorous attention to temperance as a lifestyle (for a good healer must be healthy and pure in mind and body)[47], and one which could also be usefully combined with a variety of other non-regular therapies (or with other self-helping philosophies, such as phrenology)[48]. Once again, then, as with homoeopathy, hydropathy and botanical medicine, spiritualist healing emerges as a therapeutic mode which could empower the ordinary person, and which readily forged expressive and explicit links with the political inclinations and objectives of many radicals and reformers in nineteenth century Britain.

Harrison's observation, then, that '[...] a number of Owenites and Chartists were, or later became, spiritualists, phrenologists, herbalists, vegetarians and homoeopaths'[49] is certainly true. He goes on to say that even a preliminary check of the records shows that at least ninety individuals had links with both irregular medicine and movements of social reform: further research, he suggests, would uncover more. Indeed:

> If the search were extended to include, on the one hand, involvement in education, temperance, co-operation, trade unionism, secularism, Friendly Societies and freemasonry and, on the other, anti-vaccination and physical Puritanism in general, the numbers would be even larger.[50]

Acupuncture and Osteopathy

I have attempted in the foregoing discussion, as I hope will now be clear, to account for the reasons why these connections existed, and why they appeared as such an obvious set of affiliations and allegiances to so many reformers, and to the self-improving aspirations of the many working people and artisans who supported them. Yet this network does not seem to have encompassed all

47 See the discussion of Hunt's career in Owen (1989), pp. 123–137.
48 On phrenology and self-help, see the definitive study by Cooter (1984), and also Shapin (1979), especially pp. 141–146.
49 Harrison (1987), p. 198.
50 Harrison (1987), p. 198.

of the irregular therapies which formed the web of medical pluralism in the nineteenth and early twentieth centuries. Two, in particular, merit attention and, for the sake of completeness, brief discussion: acupuncture and osteopathy.

Although the history of acupuncture in Britain can be traced as far back as the seventeenth century[51], it was not until the 1820s that any really significant medical interest in the technique can be detected, prompted largely by Churchill, a Fellow of the Royal College of Surgeons, who produced two major texts on the subject[52]. As a result of Churchill's work and further prompted by the advocacy of Elliotson – the same Elliotson who later came to professional grief because of his interest in mesmerism – acupuncture began to be taken up, albeit in a limited and sporadic way, in at least some medical quarters. For all that, it remained of marginal importance and interest to most medical men: predictably, neither the Royal College of Physicians (RCP) nor the Royal College of Surgeons were keen advocates of the technique (Dr Yates, of the RCP, called it an 'ephemeral folly').[53] This marginal status, inevitably, was not helped by the fact that acupuncture began to be plied by unlicensed practitioners, especially once the Baunschiedt device (which drove a series of spring loaded needles into the skin) became available in the 1840s. From this point onwards, acupuncture found itself included in the medical establishment's general campaign against 'quackery'; its reputation inevitably suffered, and those medical men who had taken an interest in the procedure found themselves discredited and under increasing pressure to abandon it as a therapeutic tool. Although a few isolated pockets of practice and interest remained – for example, at the Leeds Infirmary and Birmingham General Hospital[54] – the general picture, throughout the remainder of the nineteenth century and up until the 1970s, was one in which medical interest in acupuncture virtually disappeared. To all intents and purposes, it became invisible and irrelevant.[55] At the level of lay interest and activity, the story is much the same.

Why was this so? The reasons are probably not difficult to discern. Acupuncture slipped into the therapeutic backwaters probably for a number of reasons: unlike the therapies discussed above, it did not have any leading lay and/or medical advocate or advocates; it did not become a medicine for the fashionable; it was not a therapy of Anglo-European origin; it was not sufficiently transparent to be readily understood by the lay (or any other) person; it was difficult to practise; and it was embedded in a complex cosmology. Acupuncture, then, was never going to be something which could be incorporated into the self-governing and self-improving politics of the reformers and radicals in the same way as homoeopathy and its other irregular brethren.

51 Saks (1995), p. 115.
52 Churchill (1822; 1828).
53 Saks (1995), p. 117.
54 Saks (1995), p. 120.
55 Saks (1995), see especially the discussion pp. 115–133.

Osteopathy has deliberately been left for final consideration for two reasons – firstly, because it was a much later arrival on the medical scene compared to other irregular therapies and, secondly, because it was unique in its attempt to gain state recognition, and thereby to place itself on an equal legal standing with the regular profession.

One of the principal forebears of osteopathy lay in the long-standing tradition of bone-setting. Located and practising mainly in rural areas, and often on just a part-time basis, bone-setters had continued to function into the early twentieth century. Some were itinerant; others worked as part of a family tradition – and among these latter were some who acquired considerable reputations and substantial practices in the nineteenth century.[56] For the most part, bone-setters had practised without undue interference or criticism from the regular profession, although there were some exceptions, as Evan Thomas, a Liverpool practitioner, found to his cost.[57] On the whole, however, tolerance seemed to prevail – not least because bone-setting was empirical practice pure and simple, and did not seek to promote any kind of rival medical cosmology to which the medical establishment could take exception. Indeed, following John Paget's clinical lecture 'On the Cases that Bone-Setters Cure', which was published in 1867[58], a process of appropriation of the manipulative techniques which setters used to relieve dislocated, sprained or stiff joints seems to have begun as a deliberate way of adding to armoury of the developing fields of orthopaedic and physical medicine[59].

However, once Andrew Taylor Still (1828–1917) had reformulated manipulative medicine into a distinctive therapeutic modality – osteopathy – with a particular theory of the origins of disease (in the appearance of lesions in body tissues, particularly the spinal vertebrae) and its appropriate treatment, which contested the prevailing paradigm of orthodox medicine, battle was to be joined.

In the early years of the twentieth century a group of graduates from the college which Still had established in Kirksville, Missouri, had come to England where they founded, in 1911, the British Osteopathic Association. This was soon joined by a further organisation – The Incorporated Association of Osteopaths – which appeared in 1926, and to which 'untrained' (i.e. non-Kirksville trained) practitioners belonged.

It is at this point that the story becomes particularly interesting, for both organisations began to press for governmental recognition – i.e. for state registration – which would have put them on the same legal footing as the regular profession. While a variety of occupations supplementary to medicine had been successful in the quest for registration (midwives in 1902, nurses in 1919, and dentists in 1921), this had only been achieved because of the ready and willing consent of each to the dominant position of doctors in organising and

---

56   Cooter (1987), p. 160.
57   Cooter (1987), p. 163.
58   Paget (1867).
59   Cooter (1987), p. 163.

over-seeing the medical division of labour. Other supplementary occupations, like chiropodists, physiotherapists and radiographers, were willing to conclude the same bargain: occupational protection backed by the state in return for submission to medical hegemony. The osteopaths, however, did not, to use Larkin's term, wish to enlist 'medical patronage' as a mode of advancing their cause.[60] Instead, osteopaths '[…] saw themselves as having equal rights to practise in a full sense, embracing diagnosis and treatment based upon different principles of injury and healing'.[61]

The osteopaths, of course, were placing themselves in direct competition with the orthodox specialisms of orthopaedic and physical medicine, and concern with this perceived intrusion into occupied professional space begins to be seen in the language used by medical journals towards the end of the 1920s.[62] It was, however, a struggle from which the osteopaths could, at this point, never really hope to emerge victorious. By this time, the strategic alliance of medical and political power (the British Medical Association and the Ministry of Health) had become well established, and the resulting grip of the profession over healing practices and the associated medical division of labour had been progressively tightened. Certainly, as far as Ministry officials were concerned – themselves largely medically trained – the protection of improved standards of medical education and practice was intimately connected to preventing any other therapeutic group from gaining any kind of state recognition. It was the political mobilisation of this view which had defeated the Medical Herbalists' Bill in 1923; it was this same view which defeated the first Osteopaths' Registration Bill in 1931; and it was, in essence, this same view again which ensured the failure of a further registration bill for the osteopaths, introduced into the House of Lords, in 1934.

To be sure, in mounting their campaign for registration, the osteopaths had been hampered by two strategic weaknesses – uncertainty as to whether osteopathy was an 'alternative' or a 'complementary' system of medicine, and uncertainty over its therapeutic scope and range. The outcomes of their efforts, however, were to have far reaching effects, albeit certainly not the ones intended: their campaign had only served to strengthen the prevailing medical-Ministry alliance. In short, the osteopaths had provided an opportunity for medical elites to practise and hone their parliamentary strategies in defence of medical privilege. The outcome was, as Larkin points out, that '[…] heterodox practitioners in general were more easily excluded from the ensuing planning process for the National Health Service'.[63]

---

60 Larkin (1992), p. 114.
61 Larkin (1992), p. 114.
62 Larkin (1992), p. 115.
63 Larkin (1992), p. 123.

The dominance of the regular profession

The arrival of osteopathy in Britain, and its subsequent claim for state recognition, was really the last gasp of heterodox medicine's challenge to the dominance of the regular profession. The therapeutic systems which had arisen in the early decades of the nineteenth century as rivals to allopathic theory and practice were all in a process of decline by its closing decades. Homoeopathy had lost its energy, and had become introverted and even eccentric: its physicians became little more than a privileged gentleman's club catering for the rich[64] (although its continuing patronage by the Royal Family was eventually to ensure that it was the only alternative medicine to be included in plans for the National Health Service). Hydropathy eventually relinquished its claim to therapeutic distinctiveness, together with its more heroic treatments, and was easily absorbed into the repertoire of the new areas of physical, orthopaedic and rehabilitative medicine.[65] Mesmerism followed a similar route – it became respectable as hypnotism, and once this had been sanctioned as a legitimate therapeutic technique by the regular profession, the process of incorporation was well-nigh complete.[66] Spiritualism also waned, not least because new economic opportunities began to open up for the many women who had been its main practitioners.[67] As a practice, it witnessed what was probably an inevitable revival after the end of the Great War as the bereaved sought to find comfort in 'contact' with those they had lost. However, as a therapeutic modality, spiritualism began to migrate to the churches, where Christ, of course, rather than benevolent spirits in general, was seen as the source of healing power.[68] Botanical medicine, meanwhile, already weakened by internal disputes and schisms, began to look, in a modern, industrialised and urban society, as an historical relic, as part, perhaps, of what Marx had once described as 'the idiocy of rural life'.[69]

By the early decades of the twentieth century, then, the heyday of medical pluralism had certainly passed. As something in which medical men were interested, or wanted to practise, it was to all intents and purposes invisible. This is not to say that lay healers of various kinds had disappeared, as the 1910 'Report as to the Practice of Medicine and Surgery by Unqualified Persons in the United Kingdom' clearly demonstrated.[70] But such healers now really were 'a fringe': successive amendments to the Medical Act of 1858 had progressively limited what they could say, claim or do, with whom they could work, and how they could earn a living.

64 See the discussion in Nicholls (1988), especially Part IV, and also in Nicholls (1996; 2001; 2002).
65 Price (1981), see especially p. 279.
66 See the discussion in Parssinen (1979), pp. 115–117.
67 See Owen (1989), pp. 2–3.
68 See the discussion by Mews (1982).
69 See Miley/Pickstone (1988), especially pp. 150–152; and the discussion in Griggs (1981), especially chapters 18–19, 21.
70 Anon. (1910).

Why had this decline occurred? Firstly, and most obviously, because the popularity and successes of systems of medicine which had tried to incorporate the healing power of Nature into their therapeutic philosophies had had the immediate effect of weaning the regular profession away from heroic therapy. One of the key factors which had driven public sympathy for heterodox medicine was, then, beginning to disappear from even around the middle decades of the century. Secondly, the regular profession itself underwent a profound transformation during the second half of the nineteenth century: the huge expansion of hospital medicine, by weakening patient control, had created a basis for scientific innovation and, crucially, the laboratory investigation of morbid changes in body tissues.[71] It was still, of course, to be some time before effective remedies appeared that were capable of combating the pathological organisms which came, as a consequence, to be established as the necessary cause of infectious disease (the first was Salvarsan in 1910, but it was not until the sulphonamide drugs, which began to appear from 1935 onwards, and then with the wider availability of penicillin in the 1940s, that any real progress on this front was made). However, medicine's public reputation began to grow as a consequence, hospitals were no longer places to be feared, and doctors did a great deal less damage. These theoretical changes and therapeutic developments were ones with which the regular profession's old rivals could not easily compete without relinquishing much of what had been distinctive in their core philosophies in the first place. Thirdly, the political grip of the regular profession over the field of medical practice and the medical division of labour had progressively tightened – on the one hand, through developing strategic connections with the machinery of state power and, on the other, through exercising precise control over medical training (or, more technically, the means of reproduction of medical knowledge). This ensured that all graduating doctors worked with the same therapeutic paradigm. In turn, this meant, inevitably, that the identity of the medical 'other' was underscored – i.e. those (nearly all lay) practitioners whose knowledge had to be suspect and/or dangerous, and who thus needed to be shunned by the state, doctors, friendly societies, local government, and the public in general. Fourthly, the growing power of the regular profession was matched by the further development of the pharmaceutical industry. Doctors could now prescribe drugs on whose quality, strength and field of action they could rely. Although this was later to be an innovation which would lead to iatrogenic consequences at a number of levels, as Illich[72] long ago pointed out, at the time it simplified the business of doctoring, and took much of the hard work (and responsibility) out of being a patient.

As these scientific, professional and economic developments progressively ate away at the sources of heterodox medicine's popularity, so other changes in the social and political climate of the times simultaneously weakened the reform movements which had been united in the wish to bring greater self-

71 Jewson (1974; 1976).
72 Illich (1977).

determination to working people. Radical individualism might have been an appropriate way of achieving self-improvement and self-governance in earlier phases of industrialisation, but as more democratic and class based institutions strengthened and established themselves in the form of trades unions and political parties, and as the early apparatus of a state sponsored welfare system took shape, it began to appear that the optimum way of securing the betterment of ordinary people's lives within the new formations of the capitalist state would be via collective means. As the twentieth century dawned alternative therapies, which had once been natural vehicles for self-improving and self-governing lifestyles, were in headlong retreat; simultaneously, the collectively based institutions which represented the interests of a more secularised working class were becoming more established. The connection, then, was broken. Self-improvement was now to be achieved much more by class and collectively based organisations and initiatives than it was by individual effort alone, and alternative medical movements had withered in the face of a more confident, more powerful and more effective medical establishment.

It was not until the 1970s that the contours of a new post-industrial society would reconfigure in such a way that interest in non-conforming life-styles and in the celebration of counter-culture, would reignite the dialectic of change and make sense, once again, of the link between social and political radicalism, self-governance, and alternative therapy.

Bibliography

Anon.: Report as to the Practice of Medicine and Surgery by Unqualified Persons in the United Kingdom. London 1910.

Barrow, Logie: Anti-Establishment Healing: Spiritualism in Britain. In: Sheils, W[illiam] J. (ed.): The Church and Healing. (=Studies in Church History 19) Oxford 1982, pp. 225–247.

Brown, P.S.: Herbalists and Medical Botanists in Mid-Nineteenth-Century Britain with Special Reference to Bristol. In: Medical History 26 (1982), pp. 405–420.

Brown, P.S.: Social Context and Medical Theory in the Demarcation of Nineteenth-Century Boundaries. In: Bynum, W[illiam] F.; Porter, Roy (eds.): Medical Fringe and Medical Orthodoxy 1750–1850. Beckenham 1987, pp. 216–233.

Churchill, J[ames]: A Treatise on Acupuncturation. London 1822.

Churchill, J[ames]: Cases Illustrative of the Immediate Effects of Acupuncturation. London 1828.

Claridge, Richard T.: Hydropathy; or, the Cold Water Cure, as Practised by Vincent Priessnitz, at Graefenberg, Silesia, Austria. 3rd ed. London 1842.

Coffin, A[lbert] I[saiah]: A Botanic Guide to Health, and the Natural Pathology of Disease. 5th ed. Manchester 1846.

Cooter, Roger: The Cultural Meaning of Popular Science – Phrenology and the Organisation of Consent in Nineteenth-Century Britain. Cambridge 1984.

Cooter, Roger: Bones of Contention? Orthodox Medicine and the Mystery of the Bone-Setter's Craft. In: Bynum, W[illiam] F.; Porter, Roy (eds.): Medical Fringe and Medical Orthodoxy 1750–1850. Beckenham 1987, pp. 158–173.

Griggs, Barbara: Green Pharmacy. London 1981.

Gully, James: The Water Cure in Chronic Disease [...]. London 1846.

Harrison, J. F. C.: Early Victorian Radicals and the Medical Fringe. In: Bynum, W[illiam] F.; Porter, Roy (eds.): Medical Fringe and Medical Orthodoxy 1750–1850. Beckenham 1987, pp. 198–200.

Illich, Ivan: Limits to Medicine. Harmondsworth 1977.

Jewson, N[icholas]: Medical Knowledge and the Patronage System in Eighteenth Century England. In: Sociology 8 (1974), pp. 369–385.

Jewson, N[icholas]: The Disappearance of the Sick Man from Medical Cosmology 1770–1870. In: Sociology 10 (1976), pp. 225–244.

Kuhn, Thomas S.: The Structure of Scientific Revolutions. Chicago 1962.

Larkin, Gerald: Orthodox and Osteopathic Medicine in the Inter-War Years. In: Saks, Mike (ed.): Alternative Medicine in Britain. Oxford 1992, pp. 112–123.

Mews, Stuart: The Revival of Spiritual Healing in the Church of England 1920–26. In: Sheils, W[illiam] J. (ed.): The Church and Healing. (=Studies in Church History 19) Oxford 1982, pp 299–331.

Miley, Ursula; Pickstone, John V.: Medical Botany around 1850: American Medicine in Industrial Britain. In: Cooter, Roger (ed.): Studies in the History of Alternative Medicine. Basingstoke 1988, pp. 140–154.

Nicholls, Phillip A.: Homoeopathy and the Medical Profession. Beckenham 1988.

Nicholls, Phillip A.; Morrell, Peter: Laienpraktiker und häretische Mediziner: Großbritannien. In: Dinges, Martin (ed.): Weltgeschichte der Homöopathie. München 1996, pp. 185–213.

Nicholls, Phillip A.: The Social Construction and Organisation of Medical Marginality. In: Jütte, Robert et al. (eds.): Historical Aspects of Unconventional Medicine. Sheffield 2001, pp. 163–181.

Nicholls, Phillip A.: Class, Status and Gender: Toward a Sociology of the Homoeopathic Patient in Nineteenth Century Britain. In: Dinges, Martin (ed.): Patients in the History of Homoeopathy. Sheffield 2002, pp. 141–156.

Nicholls, Phillip A.: The Dialectic of the Hospital in the History of Homoeopathy. In: Medizin, Gesellschaft und Geschichte 28 (2010), pp. 281–302.

Nicolson, M[alcolm]: The Metastatic Theory of Pathogenesis and the Professional Relations of the Eighteenth Century Physician. In: Medical History 32 (1988), pp. 277–300.

Owen, Alex: The Darkened Room – Women, Power, and Spiritualism in Late Nineteenth Century England. London 1989.

Paget, James: On the Cases that Bone-Setters Cure. In: British Medical Journal (5th January 1867), pp. 1–4.

Palfreman, Jon: Between Scepticism and Credulity: A Study of Victorian Scientific Attitudes to Modern Spiritualism. In: Wallis, Roy (ed.): On the Margins of Science: The Social Construction of Rejected Knowledge. (=Sociological Review Monograph 27) Keele 1979, pp. 201–236.

Parssinen, Terry M.: Professional Deviants and the History of Medicine: Medical Mesmerists in Victorian Britain. In: Wallis, Roy (ed.): On the Margins of Science: The Social Construction of Rejected Knowledge. (=Sociological Review Monograph 27) Keele 1979, pp. 103–120.

Pickstone, John V.: Medical Botany (Self-Help Medicine in Victorian England). In: Memoirs of the Manchester Literary and Philosophical Society 119 (1976/77), pp. 85–95.

Pickstone, John V.: Establishment and Dissent in Nineteenth-Century Medicine: An Exploration of some Correspondence and Connections between Religious and Medical Belief-Systems in Early Industrial England. In: Sheils, W[illiam] J. (ed.): The Church and Healing. (=Studies in Church History 19) Oxford 1982, pp. 165–189.

Porter, Dorothy; Porter, Roy: Patient's Progress – Doctors and Doctoring in Eighteenth-Century England. Cambridge 1989.

Porter, Roy: Before the Fringe: 'Quackery' and the Eighteenth-Century Medical Market. In: Cooter, Roger (ed.): Studies in the History of Alternative Medicine. Basingstoke 1988, pp. 1–27.

Porter, Roy: Health for Sale – Quackery in England 1660–1850. Manchester 1989.

Price, Robin: Hydropathy in England 1840–70. In: Medical History 25 (1981), pp. 269–280.

Rankin, Glynis: Professional Organisation and the Development of Medical Knowledge: Two Interpretations of Homoeopathy. In: Cooter, Roger (ed.): Studies in the History of Alternative Medicine. Basingstoke 1988, pp. 46–62.

Rees, Kelvin: Water as a Commodity: Hydropathy in Matlock. In: Cooter, Roger (ed.): Studies in the History of Alternative Medicine. Basingstoke 1988, pp. 28–45.

Saks, Mike: Professions and the Public Interest – Medical Power, Altruism and Alternative Medicine. London 1995.

Sampson, Marmaduke B.: Homoeopathy: Its Principle, Theory and Practice. London 1845.

Shapin, Steven: The Politics of Observation: Cerebral Anatomy and Social Interests in the Edinburgh Phrenology Disputes. In: Wallis, Roy (ed.): On the Margins of Science: The Social Construction of Rejected Knowledge. (=Sociological Review Monograph 27) Keele 1979, pp. 139–178.

Smedley, John: Practical Hydropathy (enlarged ed.). London 1858.

Wesley, John: Primitive Physick: or an Easy and Natural Method of Curing most Diseases. First published anonymously 1747. Reprinted as: Primitive Remedies by John Wesley. Santa Barbara 1975.

Wilson, James: The Water-Cure; its Principles and Practice. London; Malvern 1857.

Medical Pluralism in France (19th to early 20th century)

Arnaud Baubérot

Introduction

The matter of medical pluralism in 19th-century and early 20th-century France may seem, at first glance, ever so slightly removed from the history of medicine – after all, this particular era opens with the law of Ventôse an XI (March 1803) offering the monopoly in healthcare to the holders of a degree in medicine. Due to this regulation that remained unchallenged throughout the six political regimes that followed, the government appeared to recognize as the only form of valid and legitimate practice of medicine that which was performed by professionals trained in the academic setting established by the state itself. As a direct consequence, all public policies regarding health and hygiene in the 19th century were designed and implemented by physicians who were medical school graduates.

Moreover, the social history of medicine in France was until recently based on the paradigm of medicalization as established by the pioneering work of Jacques Léonard.[1] The medicalization of 19th-century French society was understood as the advent of a medical profession that had control over both what was known and what was done, and could thus convert the people to their norms and practices. The growing number of physicians and their new social prestige testify to the increasing trust they gained, and the support for their view of disease and health. In spite of the reservations voiced by Léonard himself[2], the medical history of the 19th century could then be described as the gradual victory of conventional medicine over more ancient systems of therapy which were gradually silenced.

It should finally be noted that between the early 19th century and the mid-20th century, none of the medical systems formed in competition with, or in opposition to conventional medicine was able to be widespread or visible enough to represent a real danger to it. In addition, the Catholic Church, which alone in France had the institutional power to impose a divergent representation of health and disease, was far from defending a single, focused position on the matter, and never opposed any serious resistance to the emerging monopoly in care and prevention.

After all this, one could be led to read the history of medical pluralism in contemporary France as the history of a defeat suffered due to the emergence of a modern, scientific and technical medicine, always more efficient and more confident in its legitimacy. Yet, a number of factors appear to make a case for

---

1   Léonard (1981).
2   Léonard (1992), pp. 63–82.

a study of medical pluralism that is not to be confined to the chronicle of rear-guard action, but a matter that is very much relevant for the entire period.

It is first important to consider, with Patrice Bourdelais and Olivier Faure, that far from being imposed onto society by physicians, medicalization was the result of a negotiation that involved compromises.[3] Patients may have adopted the norms and methods of conventional medicine while including them into a variety of health care practices; turning to a physician could become the general rule, but not the only way, and the development of alternative therapies may have benefited from the limited efficiency of medical science.

It must also be remembered that the medical world itself was never uniform or unanimous. Beyond the debates inside academia, there are numerous examples of physicians joining non-conventional systems, and becoming agents of medical pluralism. Lastly, emphasis should be placed on the fact discussed below that from the early 19th through the mid-20th century, alternative therapeutic systems, invented and promoted by non-physicians, appeared continuously and, with varying degrees of success, tried to establish themselves in France.

The constitution of a medical power in France

In many respects, the situation of medicine and medical practitioners in 19th-century French society seems fragile and still uncertain. Firstly, the training of medical professionals was uneven, and often incomplete. While the law of 1803 admittedly granted degree holders the exclusive right to perform medical acts, those graduates were divided into two groups of unequal qualification. The first group was that of the doctors of medicine, who earned a costly degree after four years of study in one of the three medical schools of the country, in Paris, Montpellier or Strasbourg (each reclaiming in 1808 the Ancien Régime name of Faculté). They mostly had a practice in the city, and offered their services to those able to afford their fees. Those with less money and the rural population turned to the more basic care administered by health officers. These officers followed a three year program in a secondary school of medicine, following which they were accredited by a regional jury. In addition to these two groups there were the practitioners trained under the Ancien Régime as well as all those who, as the revolutionary period liberalized the practice of medicine, started calling themselves doctors and were able to obtain, without too much difficulty, authorization from the préfet to set up practice.

Still, physicians remained rare and expensive in rural France. In addition, the cultural gap between them and the population made the use of their services unpleasant. The population therefore preferred the services of healers, bone-setters and practitioners of local forms of folk medicine whose activities

---

3   Bourdelais/Faure (2005), p. 15.

were actively ignored by the authorities. The same applied to priests and nuns who recommended prayers, crucifixes or holy pictures. There was strong popular support for these forms of traditional medicine – the few lawsuits against such healers ended with a victorious physician booed by the audience as he left the court.[4]

It would however be a mistake to consider the profusion of caregivers in the French countryside of the first half of the 19th century an obstacle to its medicalization. It was rather a step in the process that reflected the decline of self-medication practices and the growing desire to consult a specialized therapist in order to maintain or regain good health. Paying more attention to results than to degrees, this population did not see the acts of healers as being against but as being complementary to a conventional medicine that was often distant and difficult to access. The public authorities, more likely to turn a blind eye to the medical acts of unsanctioned therapists than to repress them, preferred to authorize the *de facto* pluralism, as it offered a globally satisfying way to meet the demand for health care as well as access to providers.[5] The Catholic Church itself showed an ambivalent attitude. Still carried by the wave of renewed influence after the dark years of the Revolution, it encouraged religious interpretations of diseases as well as devotion to the healer saints. But at the same time, the numerous congregations of nuns bringing prayers and comfort to the sick often acted as intermediaries between them and physicians. They reported on the development of symptoms, made sure that prescriptions were followed and, when necessary, provided free medications.[6]

In terms of therapy, the boundary between the practice of degree holders and healers still remained ill-defined. With poor clinical training, physicians often considered diseases through the prism of ancient dogmas, such as the Hippocratic theory of crises, and looked for signs of its evolution in the patients' urine or perspiration. Furthermore, the pharmaceutical arsenal at their disposal was still limited, inefficient, and sometimes dangerous. Health officers practising in rural areas generally distrusted the drugs that they didn't have time to study in detail and that they found too costly for their clientele.[7] Rather than torment their patients with costly, unreliable remedies, a good number of physicians gave in to the prevalent scepticism and contented themselves with bloodletting, poultices and herbal infusions, as well as hygiene and dietary recommendations, in order to encourage the healing power of nature. The academic world itself shared this view on the traditional *materia medica*: a number of dissertations defended before 1830 praised the benefits of the *natura medicatrix* and supported, against the recklessness of aggressive therapies, the wisdom and prudence of "expectant medicine".[8]

4   Léonard (1992), p. 69.
5   Faure (1993), pp. 13–20.
6   Faure (1993), pp. 32–33.
7   Léonard (1977), pp. 54–55.
8   Baubérot (2004), pp. 30–41.

It was not until the mid-19th century that conventional medicine really began to strengthen its position. The success of medical schools resulted in a congestion of the trade, with direct effects on the population that led physicians to organize themselves against the competition of unsanctioned therapists. The "medical crowding" that physicians had pointed at since the mid-1830s should however be considered with care. It is estimated that in the mid-40s, there were about 18,000 physicians with medical degrees (10,000 doctors and 8,000 health officers), or one physician for every 1,700 inhabitants.[9] Even if one accounts for regional disparities, this is a relatively low figure. In reality, the problem of medical overpopulation was less the result of an overabundant supply of caregivers than that of low demand and a fairly narrow "medical market" owing to the limited finances of a large part of the population. For this reason, it was within the lower class, in the poorer rural regions and in the suburbs of industrial cities, that the competition of the clergy and the healers offering free or cheap care was felt the most. In 1845, the Congrès Médical de Paris underlined the need to fight the illegal practice of medicine through a rigorous organization of the medicalization of the poor.[10] The association of French physicians, AGMF (Association générale des médecins de France), founded in 1856 in continuity of the Congrès Médicaux, followed the same strategy. As an instrument of the organization and unification of the medical profession, the AGMF established itself as a weapon leading the first offensive against alternative medicine.

If physicians were able to fight such a battle in the 1860s, it was also because of the way they saw their discipline and their role in society undergo changes. The influence of positivism on the life sciences and the new paradigms introduced to the medical realm by the experimental physiology of François Magendie and later Claude Bernard, took it into the field of scientific knowledge. The observation of the succession of external symptoms, attributed to the works of a medicating nature, continually gave way to a laboratory medicine, intent on peering into the body, willing to lean close to the living organs in order to establish, through the contributions of chemistry, the principles regulating the complex mechanisms of life. Moreover, the development of scientism and faith in progress gave new strengths to the conviction of physicians. Backed by scientifically gained knowledge, armed with a more efficient therapeutics, they could now see themselves as the missionaries of "medical truth", having to carry out the sacred duty of leading the masses towards a new salvation: hygiene and health. From then on, the fight against healers was much less about defending a degree than about fending off obscurantism and heterodox doctrines.

Starting in the 1880s, the new republican power provided active support in this endeavour, for ideological as well as political reasons. At first the republican politicians shared the faith physicians had in progress and the value of scientific knowledge. Medicine then appeared as one of the practical means

9   Faure (1994), p. 100.
10   Léonard (1992), p. 67.

for science to effectively improve the living conditions of the population. But the medical community was also part of the "new social strata" that republicans had chosen to address to make it the social basis of the new regime. Indeed, physicians started to find their place in the circles of influence and the institutions of the new Republic. They could be found among radical leaders, prominent republicans – Paul Bert, Clemenceau, Emile Combes –, among the dignitaries of the Freemasons, or at the head of large cities, like Antoine Gailleton, mayor of Lyons from 1881 to 1900. In parliament, they were the second most important occupational group in the 1890s. Their political action delineated the ambitions of the regime on the issues of health and hygiene, and laid the foundation for a medical power that remained unchallenged for almost a century.

The success of the medical establishment was all the more comprehensive because there was no institutional force opposing it. A comparison with policies regulating the school system, implemented at the same time by the republicans, and the resistance against them, is particularly telling. Like the healing of bodies, the education of children was seen by the progressive elites of the 19th century as a major issue in the march towards progress. In their view, they both needed to be saved from obscurantism and placed in the care of science and reason, which meant, in the French context, that they had to be taken from the hands of the Catholic Church. Between 1881 and 1886, republican governments proposed a series of laws making primary school mandatory while secularizing public schools along with their teachers, administrators and programs. The opposition of the Church, backed by the conservative representatives, could not prevent the laws from being passed. However, despite the demands of the radical left, the laws did not give the state a monopoly on education. This educational pluralism not only allowed Catholic schools to establish themselves as a competing educational institution, but also maintained, for the bourgeoisie, the possibility of home-schooling children with the help a of a private tutor, a relatively common practice at the time. In both cases, teachers may not have had the same qualifications as the professors of the public schools. The assessment of their skills was left to the discretion of parents or head teachers. In the case of medicine, the situation was dramatically different. The republican administration put the monopoly into practice and began to impose the medical obligation through preventive hygiene or vaccination policies without meeting with any real opposition. The Catholic Church, for example, despite a few local confrontations, accepted with minimal resistance the secularization of hospitals and the requirement of a nursing degree for all nuns acting as caregivers. Two reasons can be proposed to explain this: on the one hand, the Catholic Church, having offered very little resistance to the emergence of conventional medicine throughout the century, came to accept the legitimacy of its monopoly. On the other hand, unlike the monopoly in education, the medical monopoly did not go against the practices of the upper class who could have consulted with an unconventional therapist but never treated the relationship as an element defining their social status. Equipped with this double tacit agreement, the medical power could, by the end of the 19ᵗʰ century, fully establish its hold over the medicalization of French society.

The failure of alternative systems

Another feature specific to the situation of medicine in France is that no competing system really ever threatened conventional medicine. This can be illustrated by the case of the two hydrotherapy systems designed in the 1820s by the Silesian farmer Vincenz Priessnitz and the Bavarian priest Sebastian Kneipp around 1850. Both started off as local healers with traditional methods. However, they both gained unprecedented reputation that quickly spread beyond country borders. Success led the two men to perfect their systems, and to create institutions that would soon offer care to hundreds, then thousands of patients, and serve as models for similar institutions in Europe and the United States. Associations were created in several countries which aimed at popularizing their methods and at convincing the public authorities to accredit the therapist who wished to implement them.[11]

In France, the barriers erected by the law of 1803 had two consequences in this respect. Firstly, while the relative tolerance of the government allowed healers to exercise their trade in impunity, practitioners of folk medicine were forced by the law to a certain degree of discretion. For all their success and popularity, caregivers without an official degree could not become known beyond a very local level. Therefore, no examples are known of 19ᵗʰ-century French healers who invented a new therapeutic system or were able to institutionalize their practices. Secondly, at the time when the success of the two German empirical therapists started to become known and to be followed in France, only physicians holding a degree were able to import and attempt to create any sort of institutional framework for their methods.

Priessnitz's hydrotherapy was presented for the first time in France by a young medical student, Louis Fleury, in the *Archives générales de médecine*, in 1837. In his article, Fleury underlined the therapeutic benefits of the method as well as the welcome it had received from the Austrian and German nobility. Following the article, several books by French physicians were published, all insisting on the success of hydrotherapy among the German social elites. Comforted by the prestigious endorsement, or attracted by the prospect of the fees promised by a very fashionable practice, several doctors then proceeded to create institutions of hydrotherapy. The medical overpopulation was another factor explaining the craze, as it prompted some physicians to find ways to stand out of the crowd. An additional explanation lies in the conformity of hydrotherapy to the principles of medical vitalism, still in fashion at the time. Lastly, the interest in hydrotherapy should be linked to the desire felt by a part

11 Baubérot (2004), pp. 43–53.

of the medical world to renew health care for more efficient practices. It is testament to the open-mindedness of some physicians, looking to find the future of medicine in alternative therapies. The Académie de Médecine, however, was more conservative. It condemned the Priessnitz system as early as 1840 and, in a report that reveals a corporatist defensive stance, it criticized a method "born fully clothed from the brain of a peasant" and coming "like its two elder siblings [magnetism and homeopathy], from Germany, the nebulous motherland of all great philosophical and medical impostures".[12] Despite its anti-German innuendo, the report rejected more the empiricism and unconventionality of the Priessnitz system than its origins. The presence of degree-holding physicians prescribing and supervising the care in hydrotherapy institutions eventually appeared as a necessary condition, but not sufficiently for the method to be legitimized by the medical authorities. Faced with this opposition, proponents of hydrotherapy strove, in the 1850s, to forget its naturist origins, erasing all references to *natura medicatrix* from their arguments, and to demonstrate how conform to the norms of scientific medical knowledge a treatment with cold water was. This was the case of Louis Fleury who, in his imposing 600-page "Traité pratique et raisonné d'hydrothérapie", published in 1852, contended that he wanted to "transform a medication that was potent but empirical, systematic, blind, tainted with ignorance and charlatanism, into a rational, methodical medication, acknowledged by science, in connection with the current state of our knowledge of physiology and pathology".[13] Only by stripping the method of all that characterized it as alternative medicine, and by integrating it into the field of conventional medicine, could the advocates of hydrotherapy manage to have it acknowledged as a legitimate therapy.

Faced with similar barriers, the import of homeopathy in France had a different outcome. The system designed by Hahnemann was introduced in France between the mid-1820s and the early 1830s. Unlike Priessnitz's hydrotherapy, it had not been invented by an empirical therapist, but by a physician. Its principles, however, as well as the forms of treatment it offered, made it appear as an alternative system that was at odds with the precepts of conventional medicine. A well known story is that of Sebastian des Guidi, a Neapolitan aristocrat established in Lyons, who, in 1830, founded the Société homéopathique lyonnaise. It was around him that the first dissemination networks for homeopathy in France were constituted[14]. But before that, Hahnemann's method temporarily aroused the interest also of a few physicians who would later be among the supporters of hydrotherapy. This applied to Dr Bigel from Strasbourg, for instance, who published several books, including a 3-volume treatise entitled "Examen théorique et pratique de la méthode du docteur Hahnemann, nommée homœopathie" (Warsaw 1827), before showing an interest in German hydrotherapy from 1840; it also applied to the young Louis

12 Bulletin de l'Académie royale de médecine 5 (1840), pp. 503–504.
13 On the trials and vicissitudes of hydrotherapy in France, cf. Baubérot (2004), pp. 61–80.
14 Faure (1992).

Fleury who, after his 1837 article on Priessnitz, turned for a brief period to homeopathy.[15] This suggests once more that in the medical world of the 1830s and 1840s, while the development of medicine was still hindered by the poor quality of the treatments available to official caregivers and subjected to the pressure of a society demanding more results, a minority of physicians was willing to seek solutions in the alternative systems that could demonstrate their effectiveness empirically. The development of homeopathy, which the Académie de Médecine condemned in 1835, was however relatively modest. Even thirty years later, there would only be 400 homeopaths for the entire country, less than 3% of the medical profession.[16] In addition, unlike the proponents of hydrotherapy, followers of Hahnemann in France did not seek to rewrite the justification for their system against the standards of scientific knowledge, but were content with the empirical demonstration of its effectiveness. Homeopathy therefore continued to be criticized by the medical institution, and marginalized by academia. Tolerated as long as it was practised by degree-holding physicians, it was not part, in France, of the field of conventional medicine.

Lastly, the Kneipp method was not discovered in France until the 1890s, when his German followers engaged in a strategy of worldwide communication, that included in particular the translation of the books by the Bavarian priest. They won the approval of a handful of French and Belgian priests, who in turn attempted to promote the method. They received occasional support from physicians, and a small number of hydrotherapy institutions added the "Kneipp cure" or the "Kneipp baths" to their list of services. But the vitalist arguments proposed by the Bavarian and his disciples to establish the legitimacy of the treatment were by then too outmoded to arouse any real interest from the medical community.[17]

More generally, the interest of physicians in empirical therapy systems experienced a sharp decline after the 1860s. As medicine then followed the norms of scientific knowledge, therapies had to prove their legitimacy on the basis of identifiable physiological mechanisms, in experiments that could be reproduced in a laboratory. By definition, the legitimacy of empirical systems is based solely on their ability to cure efficiently. As soon as the causes of healing must be explained, the followers of the systems in question use archaic concepts that scientific medicine no longer favours. Kneipp and his supporters claimed, for example, that all diseases were related to a corruption of humours; they referred to a "vital" or "cosmic fluid" that intervenes to restore health. Similarly, their willingness to identify the idiosyncrasies of patients stood in direct opposition to the principles of experimental medicine which seeks to establish general laws.

Yet, Louis Pasteur's discoveries gave new credibility to vitalist theories, in highlighting the ability or inability of the "terrain" to resist microbes. The idea

15   Baubérot (2004), p. 74.
16   Garden (1992), p. 69.
17   Baubérot (2004), pp. 83–95.

that natural methods could reinforce the body's defences against microbes continued to attract a number of physicians. However, these methods could only be accepted as legitimate if they give up any reference to the old notions of life force or *natura medicatrix*, and adhered at least in form, to the standards of scientific discourse.

Between the 1870s and the First World War, natural medicine was developed based on the discoveries of the physical or chemical properties of water, air and sunlight. Its supporters did not seek to expose the principles of conventional medicine, but rather to establish hydrotherapy, heliotherapy, thalassotherapy or climatotherapy within the scientific foundations, so that they could be presented as credible alternatives to chemical treatments. Grouped under the name of physiotherapy, these treatments by natural agents aroused the interest of several authorities within the medical establishment that saw them as an extension, in the therapeutic field, of their efforts to promote hygiene. For them, physiotherapy, like hygienism, took into account the decisive influence the environment has on health. Louis Landouzy, member of the Académie de Médecine, professor of therapeutics at the Faculté de Paris, and a major representative of hygienism during the Belle Epoque, made physiotherapy the topic of his 1899–1900 course. Eight years later, it was also Landouzy who welcomed inside the walls of the Faculté the first Symposium of French-speaking physicians on physiotherapy, for which he served as honorary president, a strategy that yielded mixed results, however. While physiotherapists had gained the recognition of the academic world, their procedures remained at the margin of general therapeutics. Moreover, their number was still remarkably limited – for instance, the Society of Kinesiotherapy, founded in 1900 and including practitioners of a variety of natural therapies, had only about 60 members.[18] Balneology and thermal therapies followed the same strategies and successfully established their medical legitimacy, while remaining unable to scientifically describe their positive results, by demonstrating that mineral and thermal waters brought about functional modifications. However, while integrated into the arsenal of official therapies, water therapies were reserved for the pathologies that conventional treatments were unsuccessful in curing – chronic diseases, skin and nervous disease.[19]

Permanence and renewal of alternative medicine

The clearly dominant position occupied by official medicine did not prevent unconventional treatments from persisting throughout the 19th and the first half of the 20th century. However, these therapies often followed indirect routes in order to avoid direct confrontation with the medical establishment.

Firstly, on the religious front, while the Catholic Church opposed no contest of the establishment of the medical power, it reaffirmed its vocation as a

18   Baubérot (2004), pp. 114–116.
19   Weisz (1990) and Weisz (1999), pp. 298–300.

purveyor of cures and health care operating outside the realm of science. The 19th century indeed appears as the century of healing miracles. The apparitions of the Virgin Mary in La Salette in 1846, then in Lourdes in 1858, and the miracles that followed, as well as the healings attributed to saints such as the *curé* of Ars, all invoked popular devotion that the Church made sure to encourage. Similarly, in times of epidemics, pilgrimages, processions and public prayers became more and more frequent, under the less than approving gaze of the political authorities. It was as if Catholicism was reacting to the triumph of positivism and experimental medicine by affirming the primacy of the spiritual in the health of soul and body alike. Nevertheless, the Catholic Church was very careful, throughout the 19th century, not to enter into a frontal conflict with the medical institution. Catholic physicians and the numerous nuns still active within hospitals were also means of action and channels of influence on the medical world. In addition, by entrusting the control of miraculous healings to physicians (within the Medical Bureau after 1892) before they were examined by the Church, it offered a *de facto* acknowledgment of the primacy of the medical authority when it came to health.[20]

The continuous strong tradition of self-medication also contributed to the persistence of various forms of alternative medicines. While self-medication often relied on traditional knowledge and practices transmitted within families and rural communities, it nonetheless underwent partial renewal. The development of printed media in the 19th century, as a result of both lower manufacturing costs and a higher literacy rate, made medical knowledge more accessible to the layman. A variety of "Almanacs" and "Health Manuals" offered advice on how readers could cure themselves in a way that followed the standards of conventional medicine. It was a channel that was also used to spread much less orthodox medical conceptions. It was due to this development that the books of Dr François-Vincent Raspail, published in the 1840s and advocating the virtues of a systematic use of camphor or, half a century later, the French translation of "Das neue Heilverfahren" ("The New Natural Medication", Paris 1898) by Friedrich Eduard Bilz became such a great success. Furthermore, their enthusiasm for medications and remedies drove the French to indiscriminately purchase, most of the time without a prescription, conventional drugs designed by accredited pharmacists as well as the most exotic pills and elixirs.[21]

Self-medication is also the channel through which the care system invented by Kneipp finally reached a French clientele. Starting in the 1890s, Joseph Favrichon, a pharmacist in Saint-Symphorien-de-Lay in Loire, and Emile Burrel, an entrepreneur from Lyons, started a mail-order business supplying hygiene and care products manufactured after the recommendations of the Bavarian priest, such as flax yarn shirts, malt coffees, vegetable-based hair pomades, elixirs, plant-based salves. Two significant distribution networks were created, soon to be at odds with one another. One of them, called Favri-

---

20 Guillaume (1990).
21 Faure (1993), pp. 62–68.

chon, supplied 19 bakeries and 13 trading firms, among them "La méthode Kneipp", a Parisian store specialized in trading naturist goods. The other, Burrel's Institution Kneipp de France, supplied 34 bakeries and 25 grocery stores. In 1897, the institution opened its own retail outlet in Lyons, and gained the monopoly on the commercial use of the name Kneipp in France. These two examples, in the context of the dramatic increase of hygiene and dietetics stores in the major cities of France, underline the rapid growth of new health practices at the medical fringe.[22]

The same trend is also reflected, from the 1900s through the 1930s, in the new interest some physicians showed in the tradition of medical naturism. Similarly to the physiologists who rejected chemical treatment and preferred natural therapies, they differed in their condemnation of conventional medicine, and their refusal to adhere to its standards. They did not hesitate to explicitly refer to old neo-Hippocratic or vitalist notions, or to draw from the therapeutics of the German empiricists. In terms of treatments, they abandoned cold water, used in natural medicine throughout the 19th century, advocating the use of air and sun instead. These treatments were more in keeping with the new views on lifestyle and were seen as offering help for the body to recharge its vital energy, when older methods of hydrotherapy aimed to stimulate the circulation of the vital fluid and ease the flow of humours through the application of ice-cold water. The very gentle applications of aerotherapy and heliotherapy made them all the more attractive to the hedonistic upper classes, who increasingly owned summer houses on the Mediterranean rather than on the northern shores. For example, in 1909, Dr Monteuuis left Dunkirk and his 20 year old practice of thalassotherapy at the seafront, and moved south to the Côte d'Azur. There, he set up a sanatorium, its park equipped with *huttes d'air* ("air huts" are small cabins made of three walls and a roof, open on one side), that had been invented by the Swiss empiricist Arnold Rikli and were subsequently found in many a German naturist institution. Monteuuis' patients, during their stay, took partially or fully nude "air and sun baths". Far from being an isolated case, Monteuuis' institution was one of just under 10 naturist establishments on the French Riviera.[23]

The same interest in the hygienic and curative virtues of air and sun can be found with the brothers André and Gaston Durville. They were the sons of magnetizer Hector Durville and were both doctors of medicine who followed an unconventional path from early in their career, showing interest in "magnetic medicine" and "experimental psychism". They turned to naturism in the early 1920s, and devoted the rest of their career to its study, as hygienists rather than therapists. They published a number of periodicals and books promoting naturism, and set up two resorts, one in the Paris area, the other in Var, where sports and "sun cures" were practised.

Lastly, the case of Dr Paul Carton, the main apostle of medical naturism of the inter-war period, must be mentioned. Reneging, due to anti-German senti-

22   Baubérot (2008).
23   Baubérot (2004), pp. 120–125.

ments, the benefits of empirical therapies, he strove to find in Greco-Latin sources the foundation for an alternative approach to health and healing. In more than 30 books – reprinted several times and translated into various European languages (German excluded) – he again and again condemned conventional medicine for trying hard to get rid of the symptom, and ignoring the deeper causes of diseases. For him, these causes had to be systematically sought in the diet and lifestyle that did not suit the temperament of the patient. For Carton, the role of the physician was not to administer a generic therapy, but to study the physical and mental constitution of their patients, so that a carefully thought out diet could be prescribed, and the patients could be led back to the path of healthy living.[24]

The discourse and practices of these physicians conveyed an open criticism of modern medicine. They refused to focus on the dysfunction of a diseased organ and advocated a holistic view of the human being and his relation to his environment. Beyond the technical and industrial evolution of medicine and therapeutics, their criticism was also aimed at contemporary lifestyles that, as they argued, drove people away from the laws of nature. It would not do them justice if one considered these unconventional practices and therapeutics as an outburst of nostalgia to induce those disillusioned by modernity to look back and try to revive outmoded and archaic ideas on medicine. Rather, they could be described as avatars of anti-modernism which, like all anti-modernist reactions, were integral parts of the modernity they criticized and, as such, aspects of the same modernity. Indeed, medical naturism resulted above all from the actions of physicians with an academic background, who turned to alternative therapies not because they had a nostalgic preference for the past but rather because they sought for ways of complementing a contemporary medicine that they found to be insufficient. Their effort must also be considered in the context of a more general movement seeking new social practices that would make up for the inconveniences of urban and industrial civilization, a search for diets and well-being understood to be more in harmony with nature.

Lastly, on a purely medical level, these practitioners of natural medicine are waving ancient Hippocratic notions in favour of practices that are, in effect, truly innovative. It would then stand to reason to consider that the development of modern medicine, for all the exclusiveness it claims for itself, has created the new forms of medical pluralism.

It should finally be underlined that this alternative approach to health emerged during the 20th century, in a space left empty by the modern regime of science and religion. On one hand, medical science has excluded metaphysical concerns from its realm in order to focus on the study of limited and identifiable causality that can be reproduced in a laboratory. On the other hand, in secular societies, the religious discourse renounces more and more all metaphysical explanations for health and sickness. Between the two, the ques-

24   Baubérot (2004), pp. 249–278.

tion of fundamental causes and ultimate ends is left with no other answer than chance and probabilities. Yet, patients are rarely content with those answers, and ask that meaning be given to their disease. In describing nature as an order within which human beings must find harmony, so that their health can be maintained or found again, alternative medicine offers the answer to this very question.

Bibliography

Baubérot, Arnaud: Histoire du naturisme. Le mythe du retour à la nature. Rennes 2004.

Baubérot, Arnaud: Un projet de réforme hygiénique des modes de vie: naturistes et végétariens à la Belle Époque. In: French Politics, Culture and Society 26 (2008), no. 3, pp. 1–22.

Baubérot, Jean; Liogier, Raphaël: Sacrée médecine. Histoire et devenir d'un sanctuaire de la Raison. Paris 2010.

Bourdelais, Patrice; Faure, Olivier (eds.): Les nouvelles pratiques de santé. Acteurs, objets, logiques sociales (XVIIIe–XXe siècles). Paris 2005.

Bulletin de l'Académie royale de médecine 5 (1840), pp. 503–504.

Faure, Olivier (ed.): Praticiens, patients et militants de l'homéopathie (1800–1940). Lyon 1992.

Faure, Olivier: Les Français et leur médecine au XIXe siècle. Paris 1993.

Faure, Olivier: Histoire sociale de la médecine (XVIIIe–XXe siècles). Paris 1994.

Garden, Maurice: Histoire de l'homéopathie en France, 1830–1940. In: Faure, Olivier (ed.): Praticiens, patients et militants de l'homéopathie (1800–1940). Lyon 1992, pp. 60–79.

Guillaume, Pierre: Médecins, Église et foi, XIXe-XXe siècles. Paris 1990.

Léonard, Jacques: La vie quotidienne du médecin de province au XIXe siècle. Paris 1977.

Léonard, Jacques: La médecine entre les savoirs et les pouvoirs. Histoire intellectuelle et politique de la médecine française au XIXe siècle. Paris 1981.

Léonard, Jacques: Médecins, malades et société dans la France du XIXe siècle. Paris 1992.

Weisz, George: Water Cures and Science: The French Academy of Medicine and Mineral Waters in the Nineteenth Century. In: Bulletin of the History of Medicine 64 (1990), no. 3, pp. 393–416.

Weisz, George: Stations thermales et eaux minérales dans la France du XXe siècle. In: Faure, Olivier (ed.): Les Thérapeutiques: savoirs et usages. Lyon 1999, pp. 285–301.

Medical Plurality and Medical Pluralism in Germany (19th and early 20th century)

Gunnar Stollberg

Pluralism and plurality

Medical pluralism is often discussed basing on the critical concept of a new medical pluralism as suggested by Cant and Sharma in 1999. This concept may be useful for debating today's structures and problems. But the two authors give only a few characteristics of the 'old' medical pluralism that vanished by the second half of the 19th century in Britain[1]: There was a flourishing medical market, and biomedicine had only a limited measure of advantage. Nevertheless I firstly doubt that there was a clear form of biomedicine in the first half of the 19th century. Secondly it is difficult to draw a clear difference between old and new medical pluralism, except for the fact that phenomena like professionalism, biomedicine etc. were not developed yet. Thus I suggest replacing the difference between old vs. new medical pluralism by a difference between medical plurality (or medical diversity) and medical pluralism. 'Plurality' characterises a variety of phenomena in a given social field. They do co-exist, maybe competing, maybe co-operating, and maybe ignoring each other. Actors and observers construct a social field as a unity, and observe similar phenomena co-existing in this field as plurality. For example medical anthropologists differentiated between local and regional medical systems and the cosmopolitan medical system[2], or divided health care systems in given nation states or regions into folk, popular and professional sectors[3]. Meanwhile some of them use terms like plurality[4] or plural medicine[5]. Waltraud Ernst suggests 'to differentiate carefully between the desirability of medical pluralism and the extent to which it has been realised in a "globalised" medical world that is still powerfully dominated by American and European pharmaceutical firms'[6] etc. Baer goes into the same direction stressing that 'national medical systems in the modern world tend to be "plural" rather than "pluralistic"'.[7] Indeed, it may be useful to differentiate between medical plurality and pluralism.

1 Cant/Sharma (1999), p. 194.
2 Cf. Dunn (1976).
3 Cf. Kleinman (1980).
4 Cf. Scheid (2002).
5 German medical anthropologists obviously got no problems using the term 'medical pluralism', defined as the parallel existence of Kleinman's different health care systems in a nationally defined society. Cf. Pfleiderer/Greifeld/Bichmann (1995), p. 86. Cf. already Pfleiderer/Bichmann (1985), p. 163.
6 Waltraud Ernst (2001), p. 4.
7 Baer (2004), p. 111.

What is 'pluralism'? In political philosophy, the term denotes a political order characterised by a competition of political elites, and a political bargaining of interest groups. Dahl, having recourse to Locke, enunciated a central idea of political pluralism: 'no one can be [...] subjected to the Political Power of another without his own Consent'.[8] Thus a mutual acknowledgement of the citizens' interests forms a basic principle of the pluralist democratic process. The Harvard Pluralism Project looks at world religions in the USA from a similar perspective: In contrast to a mere diversity, the dynamic of pluralism 'is one of meeting, exchange, and two-way traffic'.[9] Thus, pluralism means an active engagement with diversity or plurality; it requires some mutual knowledge of the differences. Actors and conceptions acknowledge other actors and conceptions as members of a common social field. In this sense, medical pluralism denotes an order of medical actors and conceptions acknowledging other actors and conceptions to be members of the medical system within a (national) society.

But here we have to make a difference, again. We can differentiate a politically and legally based medical pluralism from a medically based medical pluralism. The politically based medical pluralism relies on a political compromise.[10] The medically based medical pluralism bases on a mutual acknowledgment of different medical conceptions within medicine.

In my paper I will demonstrate that Germany passed from medical plurality at about 1800 to fragile forms of pluralism since the 1870s.

Medical plurality in 19th century

Let me characterise the medical plurality of the 19th century by a passage from the autobiography of the journalist Friedrich Oetker in 1878 (at that time, he was 69 years old):

> No wonder that I often encountered with physicians! Up to now, 51 have treated me in a formal manner. The number of those having examined or counselled me casually is certainly three times higher, from the students at Marburg to Oppolzer[11]; the number of sympathetics, magnetizers, spiritual healers, expert shepherds, and wise women not in-

---

8   Cf. Dahl (1989), p. 85. Locke (1966), chapter VIII, & 95.
9   Cf. Eck (2006), quoted from http://www.pluralism.org/pages/pluralism/essays/from_diversity_to_pluralism (accessed 5 December 2012).
10 Looking from systems theory, we can differentiate a medical pluralism basing on a mutual acknowledgement of medical programs from a pluralism basing on acknowledgement originating from another functional system that is structurally coupled with medicine. This is especially true for the political system. The acknowledgement within the medical system can be performed on the level of science, and/or of the profession. The acknowledgement within the political system may result from social policy and its institutions.
11 Johann Ritter von Oppolzer (1808–1871), professor of medicine in Prague, Leipzig, and since 1850 in Vienna.

cluded yet. Medicorum turba perii, said Hadrian, I think. Thank God I can say: non perii.[12]

Oetker's autobiography demonstrates that a member of the educated middle class used many healers in parallel manner from the 1820s to the 1870s. He did neither hesitate nor conceal using also various non-academic healers. Oetker mentions two heterodox medical conceptions: Mesmerism and folk medicine.[13] The physician Franz Anton Mesmer (1734–1815) proposed an animal magnetism that became effective in a bodily magnetic fluidum applied to the sick body by hand or by a stick. A Prussian royal commission acknowledged the principle, but proposed to use it only under the supervision of the authorities. In the second half of the 19th century the animal magnetism became scientifically outdated, but remained a popular practice. In science, hypnosis took its place.[14]

Folk medicine, the second heterodoxy mentioned by Oetker, is the healing technique of the rural population in contrast to scientific or professional medicine.[15] The practices of shepherds or of wise women were often accepted within the urban population, because urbanisation brought about many changes in everyday life. Folk medicine and natural healing both could use adverse reactions to these changes.

During the 19th century, the relationship between the popular and the professional medical sectors underwent some changes: In its first three decades, dietetics and self-medication were central devices of the educated middle classes. But they did not form an alternative to using healers. These healers could be folk healers, or artisan surgeons, or academic doctors. In the autobiographies stemming from members of the educated urban classes, folk healers like wise women were seen for luxations, or rheumatics. Surgeons were not called by name, while academic doctors were often integrated into ties of friendship and individuation. Surgeons and barbers were called for less dangerous health problems; academic doctors for more serious ones.[16]

By the end of the century, the device of self-medication (become your own doctor) became replaced by calling for medical specialists within the educated classes. The lay referral system was restricted to the first contacts with healers, while the doctors referred to other professionals. Following the establishment of the public health insurance system since the 1880s, the call for a thorough examination performed by an academic doctor replaced self-medication even among artisans and workers.[17] This development can be characterised as medicalisation from below.

12 Translated from Lachmund/Stollberg (1995), p. 67.
13 The second wave of the reception of acupuncture might form a third contemporary heterodox concept. Cf. Kerber (1832).
14 Cf. Jütte (1996), p. 109.
15 Cf. Kleinman (1980).
16 Cf. Lachmund/Stollberg (1995), pp. 126ff.
17 Cf. Lachmund/Stollberg (1995), p. 206.

Medical plurality can be observed on the level of individual healers and their patients, but also on the level of organisations.[18] Societies (*Vereine*) acted as intermediary institutions between individuals and society.[19] In the field of medicine, homoeopathic societies existed since the 1830s. Their association comprised some 29,000 members in 1912 and some 48,000 in 1936. Regional strongholds were industrialised regions like Wurttemberg, Saxony, the Rhineland, and Westphalia. The social structure widened from the petty bourgeoisie to industrial workers in the 1920s.

Much more members were organised by societies for natural healing (*Naturheilvereine*). The German association of societies for living and healing according to nature (*Deutscher Bund der Vereine für naturgemäße Lebens- und Heilweise*) reached a maximum number of 148,000 members in 1913.[20] The competing Kneipp societies[21] comprised 42,000 members in 1928, and some 150,000 in our times. These associations demonstrate the popularity of non-biomedical conceptions since 19th century.

Neither Mesmerism nor homoeopathy nor natural healing were conceptions of medical laypersons only. Mesmer and Hahnemann were medical doctors themselves, while Prießnitz and Kneipp were laypersons. But they attracted medical doctors to their respective environments, and these doctors transferred the water cures into medical conceptions. A medical conception is a coherent system of explanations of the body, disease, and therapy. Prießnitz was an agricultural housekeeper. His medical practices were transformed into a conception of natural healing by the dispensing chemist Theodor Hahn and the Bavarian military physician Dr Lorenz Gleich in the 1850s. Kleinschrodt and later Baumgarten, both medical doctors, assisted the parson Kneipp in his public consultation hours in the 1880s and 1890s.

Juridical developments: From regulations against quackery to the freedom of curing

We can observe medical plurality all over the 19th century, though many German cities had banned the activities of quacks (*Pfuscher*) since the 16th century.[22] In the 18th century quackery raised most concerns regarding the lack of licence.[23] The city regulations were followed by many German states since

---

18   Cf. Stollberg (1991).
19   For associations as organisations organising sociality and conviviality, cf. Nathaus (2009) and Hoffmann (2003). Both the authors do not particularly go into the societies for natural healing.
20   Cf. Regin (1995).
21   The German Association stands within the tradition of Prießnitz. Kneipp took over many points from Prießnitz, but founded a conception of his own. The Kneipp societies competed with the Prießnitz societies, and over passed them after WW II.
22   Cf. Graack (1906), pp. 6–7.
23   In late 19th century, the medical campaign against quacks (*Kurpfuscher*) attacked the lack of training and adequate medical knowledge of healers who had not attended university

the late 17th century, and even corroborated by criminal law in the 19th century. But in fact, the principle of livelihood (*bürgerliche Nahrung*), of an equitable distribution of the economic pie[24], was more important than the formal qualification of healers. It favoured non formally qualified healers.

In 1869 the North German Federation (*Norddeutscher Bund*) introduced liberal regulations concerning the freedom of curing (*Kurierfreiheit*), which were adopted by the German Reich. Every woman and every man became allowed to execute the art of healing in all its branches. But s/he was not allowed to hold the title of or similar to a doctor/physician (*Arzt*), if s/he had not successfully completed medical studies at a university.

The century from the 1850s to the 1950s can be conceptualised as being the century of the medical profession. Medicine became professionalised.[25] I give some dates for this process: In 1852 Prussia legislated for a medical profession unifying internal medicine, surgery, and obstetrics. In 1864 the state of Baden and in 1887 Prussia founded medical associations with official duties and responsibilities. By the establishment of a social health insurance system in the 1880s, physicians became gatekeepers for insurance benefits. By the 1970s, the physicians' autonomy became restrained by the development of organisational fields comprising other health occupations, and by bureaucratic regulations.[26]

I return to the liberal freedom of curing regulation in 1869. It legally transformed the academic physicians from a profession to the level of a normal business. Though it opened some advantages to the physicians – they were no longer bound to the traditional tariffs, and their collectivity was no longer in charge of the entire population –, it soon became attacked by the medical associations. They aimed at restricting healing activities to medical doctors. Though they gained some smaller victories[27], they could not end the freedom of curing[28] before the Nazi period, or even until today.

The freedom of curing was formally abolished by law in 1933; any healing occupation was restricted to physicians only. In 1939, a law regulated the healing activities of non-medical qualified personnel. Healers, who were practicing at that time, had to apply for a special licence. Persons with special healing abilities should be allowed to study at a university, without having passed the A level (*Abitur*). In its strict form, the law became effective in the German Democratic Republic only. In Western Germany, the *Heilpraktiker* were al-

---

studies.

24 Cf. Lindemann (1996), p. 165.

25 Distinguishing marks of a profession are a special area of knowledge connected with a scientific discipline, the formation of associations, and the jurisdiction in a special social field.

26 Cf. Döhler (1997).

27 Cf. Göckenjan (1987).

28 There are scarcely any exact figures about non-medically qualified healers. In 1902, Prussia obliged them to become registered. In the first year 4,104 healers were registered, 7,549 in 1908. The increase may be due to more efficient registration methods. Cf. Huerkamp (1985), p. 277.

lowed to practice when having passed a kind of examination at a local health authority.

I can summarise: The laws constraining quackery aimed at defining healers' qualification by university studies, but did not actually constrain medical plurality. The juridical development in the years between 1869 and 1933 transformed medical plurality into a legally based pluralism. The freedom of curing implied a legal and political acknowledgement of different medical conceptions. It opened the way to a politically based medical pluralism.

The peak of this development was reached by the West German pharmaceuticals act in 1976: Different commissions were established that decide on the approval of drugs. As for biomedical drugs, they differ for medical subjects. But there is a second differentiation: Homoeopathically oriented doctors form commissions for the approval of homoeopathic drugs, anthroposophical doctors for anthroposophic drugs, and phytotherapists for herbal drugs. This differentiation followed a political compromise; biomedical scientists never accepted this pluralism.[29]

Since 2004, the Federal Joint Commission produces guidelines outlining the list of services covered by the statutory health insurance. This organisation developed within the tradition of Keynesian concerted actions to reduce the costs of health services.[30] As medical scientists and (other) physicians are members of this Commission, its decisions form a mixture of politically and medically based pluralism.

Medical unity and medically based pluralism:
The development of biomedicine

Medical pluralism requires an institution of acknowledgement. On the one side, law fulfils this function. On the other side, medicine has to develop institutions of its own. Biomedicine is able to construct these institutions. But what is biomedicine? It is the reflexion theory of modern medical systems. As a reflexion theory, it defines the field and the borders of medicine. It constructs an illusion of a conceptual unity in moments when medicine is at stake. Biomedicine reflects a medical science oriented to natural sciences. Developing through 19th century, it defined itself by contrast towards competing conceptions, like homoeopathy from ca. 1810–1850, and natural healing from ca. 1850–1880.[31]

In 18th century Germany the concept of livelihood 'furnished the essential key to understanding how people constructed and perceived their identi-

29 Cf. Plagemann (1979); Kevelaer (1980).
30 The Concerted Action in the Health System had been established in 1977. In 1989, Federal Commissions of Physicians and Sickness Funds were founded. They substituted the Concerted Action functionally.
31 Cf. Jütte (1996), pp. 23–32.

ties'.[32] This was also true for the medical marketplace or field. Surgeons and physicians showed a guild mentality.[33] But livelihood often favoured non-medically qualified healers.

Since the 1830s, physicians defined medicine as a profession directed by science. In 1831, Christoph Wilhelm Hufeland (1762–1836), a medical authority of his time, councillor in the Prussian ministry of domestic affairs, claimed his medical conception to be rational – in contrast to Hahnemann's homoeopathy.[34] This harsh statement formed a late stage of the relationship between Hufeland and Hahnemann. In the years between 1801 and 1807, Hahnemann had published several articles in Hufeland's *Journal of the practical art of healing (Journal der practischen Arzneikunde)*. But above all, Hahnemann shared Hufeland's aspirations 'to create a medicine to match the real achievements of the sciences'.[35] Though Hahnemann founded his own medical conception on experience, in his books he discussed German, English, and French medical authors. Thus, the boundaries of biomedicine have been drawn arbitrarily from the very beginnings.

Biomedicine forms less a medical conception than a reflexion theory of medicine.[36] During the 19th century we can observe the development of this reflexion theory. The paradigm of humoral pathology frayed, like we can observe in Hufeland's famous 'Enchiridion medicum' (1836). There we can find a classification of diseases putting fevers, congestions and many other categories on a level parallel to the humoral dyscrasias. Conceptions strange to the Galenic tradition emerged. In the first years of the 19th century, the Romantic philosopher Friedrich Wilhelm Schelling (1775–1854), who strongly influenced the medical thought of his time, differentiated between two external worlds of the organism.[37] The inner external world consisted of the four humours of the Galenic tradition; it interfered with and reconstituted the equilibrium of the organism. Schelling's conception opened the path to biomedicine and especially to Claude Bernard's (1813–1879) concept of a milieu interieur in the 1860s.

As a second aspect of biomedicine, qualitative approaches were replaced by quantitative ones since the 1820s. Pierre Louis and Lambert Quetelet must be mentioned in this context. In Germany they were followed by Friedrich Oesterlen's 'Handbook of Medical Statistics' in 1865.[38] This scientification of medicine became clear in Josef Dietl's proclamation dating from 1845: 'Medi-

---

32 Lindemann (1996), p. 203.
33 Cf. Lindemann (1996), p. 171.
34 Cf. Jütte (1996), p. 26.
35 Dean (2004), p. 9, assumes that homoeopathy's attention to the patient's person on the one hand, and some of its streams on the other side made academic medicine exclude the homoeopathic conception.
36 In systems theory, reflexion theories are forms of the self-reflexion of functional social systems. They describe the identity of the respective functional system in a way that comparisons and correspondences may follow up; cf. Luhmann (1984), p. 620.
37 Cf. Tsouyopoulos (2008), p. 135.
38 Cf. Fangerau/Martin (2011), pp. 56–57.

cine is a science, basing on mathematics, like every science'.[39] Its status as an exact science implies that the therapies of this time got no scientific base yet, but relied on anthropology.[40] This change of the reference discipline opened the way to new techniques of medical measurement, like determining the numbers of erythrocytes in human blood[41], drawing fever charts[42] etc.

By the end of 19th century, these paths away from humoral pathology were interpreted as a clearly aligned and strong victory of biomedicine over philosophical speculation. But this interpretation did not exist yet at about 1850. For example: Since the 1890s, the encyclopaedias praised the alleged refutation of vitalism in the 1840s as a central step towards biomedicine. But in the 1840s, the protagonists did not interpret organic chemistry as a refutation of vitalism yet.[43]

I can summarise that biomedicine as a reflexion theory constructing medicine as a science represented by a profession slowly developed all along 19th century.

Medical pluralism remains restricted to the political base: The history of professorships for homoeopathy and natural healing at German universities

Seeking scientific acknowledgment, the non-biomedical conceptions aimed at establishing professorships at medical faculties. Though or because the universities formed a conservative bastion of science, a professorship would have been a clear sign of acknowledgement. Homoeopathic physicians were allowed to give lectures since the 1830s[44], but a professorship was denied. As late as 1939, Hitler named the 69 years old Ernst Bastanier, head of a university homoeopathic ambulance in Berlin, as a professor. Hanns Rabe followed in 1939, and Alfons Stiegele, head of the homoeopathic Robert-Bosch-Hospital in Stuttgart, in 1940. Homoeopathy thus did not become fully acknowl-

---

39 Cf. Tsouyopoulos (2008), p. 125. Dietl (1804–1878) was a medical doctor from Vienna.
40 Cf. Rothschuh (1978), p. 428.
41 In 1852 by Vierordt, improved by Malassais, Thoma-Zeiss and others.
42 By Carl August Wunderlich in the 1860s.
43 By the 1840s the conception of a life force demised, though it was partly compatible with physicalism. The latter became the dominant paradigm, and it constructed a myth of victory by refutation. In 1890, 'Meyers Konversations-Lexikon' (4th ed., vol. 10) praised Lotze to have refuted life force, which had been the core of vitalism, in 1842 (vol. 17). In 1990, 'Brockhaus' Enzyklopädie' (19th ed., vol. 13) dated the first refutation of life force back to 1828, when the chemist Friedrich Wöhler (1800–1882) produced the organic urea by a combination of the inorganic cyanic acid with ammonia. This myth has been unmasked since 1944; cf. Teich/Needham (1992), pp. 451–452. Wöhler and his contemporaries had not seen the preparation of urea as a refutation of vitalism.
44 Hahnemann had given lectures at Leipzig University in the years between 1812 and 1821. But his success remained limited, and only part of the lectures had homoeopathy for its topics; cf. Jütte (2005), p. 106.

edged on the university level, and had to be content with the establishment of wards and hospitals since the 1840s.

As for natural healing, Ludwig Brieger became head of the Berlin hydro-therapeutic university institute in 1901.[45] After his death in 1920, the Social Democratic Prussian minister Haenisch named Dr. med. Franz Schönenberger as a professor for natural healing. The appointment met the resistance of the faculty. After Schönenberger's death in 1933, it took a long time, till a professor for natural healing was appointed in 1989 at the Free University of (West-) Berlin. Thus the medically acknowledged pluralism remained contested up to our days.

Outlook: Steps towards a medically based medical pluralism

The medically based medical pluralism was prepared by scientific studies of the efficacy of drugs and medical practices. Such studies were practiced since the 1820s.[46] In our times, 'Evidence Based Medicine' (EBM) became an important evaluation method in many modern countries. The Scottish epidemiologist Archie Cochrane (died 1988) had propagated an evidence based medicine against the eminence based medicine of medical authorities. Meanwhile, two different streams can be observed within evidence based medicine[47]: The evidence-based support for therapeutic decisions of individual physicians, and the mainstream, the production of evidence-based guidelines. The methodological spectre reached from individual case reports to randomised clinical studies.[48] The randomised clinical trials (RCTs) have become the silver bullet in medical science, however.[49]

In 1976, the peak of politically based pluralism was reached in Western Germany with the pharmaceuticals act. In our days, the rocky road to a medically based pluralism is advanced by RCTs.[50] The partial integration of acupuncture into the list of services covered by public health insurance companies may be interpreted as such a step. From 2002 to 2005 huge randomised trials were performed. In 2006, the Federal Joint Committee could resort to their results deciding that acupuncture should be paid by public health insurance companies in cases of chronic pain in lumbar region and arthrosis of the knee. And since 2003, the Medical Associations introduced a (minor) specialisation in acupuncture for physicians.

Thus in the case of acupuncture, evidence based medicine worked at least partially in favour of a medical base of pluralism. But in the case of herbal

---

45 Brieger was an extra-ordinary professor for internal medicine and general therapy since 1890.
46 Cf. Dean (2004), pp. 101ff.
47 Cf. Eddy (2005).
48 Cf. Gerhardus (2006).
49 Cf. Edzard Ernst et al. (2001).
50 Kiene's (2001) proposition of a cognition-based medicine remained contested.

medicine, we today can observe evidence based medicine to work against this base. Medical pluralism is not a stable phenomenon, neither historically nor in our times.

Bibliography

Baer, Hans A.: Medical Pluralism. In: Ember, Carol (ed.): Encyclopedia of Medical Anthropology. Vol. I: Topics. New York et al. 2004, pp. 109–116.

Cant, Sarah; Sharma, Ursula: A New Medical Pluralism? Alternative Medicine, Doctors, Patients and the State. London 1999.

Dahl, Robert A.: Democracy and its Critics. New Haven; London 1989.

Dean, Michael Emmans: The Trials of Homeopathy. Origins, Structure and Development. Essen 2004.

Döhler, Marian: Strukturbildung von Politikfeldern. Das Beispiel bundesdeutscher Gesundheitspolitik seit den fünfziger Jahren. Opladen 1997.

Dunn, Frederick L.: Traditional Asian Medicine and Cosmopolitan Medicine as Adaptive Systems. In: Leslie, Charles M. (ed.): Asian Medical Systems. A Comparative Study. Berkeley 1976, pp. 133–158.

Eck, Diana L.: On Common Ground. World Religions in America. 2nd ed. New York 2006.

Eddy, David M.: Evidence-based Medicine: a Unified Approach. In: Health Affairs 24 (2005), pp. 9–17.

Ernst, Edzard et al. (eds.): The Desktop Guide to Complementary and Alternative Medicine. An Evidence-based Approach. Edinburgh et al. 2001.

Ernst, Waltraud (ed.): Plural Medicine. London 2001.

Fangerau, Heiner; Martin, Michael: Konzepte von Gesundheit und Krankheit: Die Historizität elementarer Lebenserscheinungen zwischen Qualität und Quantität. In: Viehöver, Willy; Wehling, Peter (eds.): Entgrenzung der Medizin. Von der Heilkunst zur Verbesserung des Menschen? Bielefeld 2011, pp. 51–66.

Gerhardus, Ansgar: Die Umsetzung von Forschung in die Praxis. In: Razum, Oliver; Zeeb, Hajo; Laaser, Ulrich (eds.): Globalisierung – Gerechtigkeit – Gesundheit. Einführung in International Public Health. Bern 2006, pp. 177–187.

Göckenjan, Gerd: Nicht länger Lohnsklaven und Pfennigkulis? Zur Entwicklung der Monopolstellung der niedergelassenen Ärzte. In: Deppe, Hans-Ulrich; Friedrich, Hannes; Müller, Rainer (eds.): Medizin und Gesellschaft. Jahrbuch 1. Frankfurt/Main; New York 1987, pp. 9–36.

Graack, Henry: Kurpfuscherei und Kurpfuschereiverbot. Eine rechtsvergleichende, kriminalpolitische Studie. Jena 1906.

Hoffmann, Stefan-Ludwig: Geselligkeit und Demokratie. Vereine und zivile Gesellschaft im transnationalen Vergleich 1750–1914. Göttingen 2003.

Huerkamp, Claudia: Der Aufstieg der Ärzte im 19. Jahrhundert. Göttingen 1985.

Jütte, Robert: Geschichte der Alternativen Medizin. München 1996.

Jütte, Robert: Samuel Hahnemann. Begründer der Homöopathie. München 2005.

Kerber, Theodorus: Dissertatio inauguralis medico-chirurgica de acupunctura. Halis Saxonum 1832.

Kevelaer, Karl-Heinz v.: Das Arzneimittelgesetz von 1976. Entstehungsbedingungen und Entscheidungsprozeß. Dipl.-Soz. Arbeit Bielefeld (MS) 1980.

Kiene, Helmut: Komplementäre Methodenlehre der Klinischen Forschung. Cognition-based Medicine. Berlin et al. 2001.

Kleinman, Arthur: Patients and Healers in the Context of Culture. An Exploration of the Borderline between Anthropology, Medicine, and Psychiatry. Berkeley 1980.

Lachmund, Jens; Stollberg, Gunnar: Patientenwelten. Krankheit und Medizin vom späten 18. bis zum frühen 20. Jahrhundert im Spiegel von Autobiographien. Opladen 1995.

Lindemann, Mary: Health & Healing in Eighteenth Century Germany. Baltimore 1996.

Locke, John: Second Treatise on Government. Oxford 1966.

Luhmann, Niklas: Soziale Systeme. Frankfurt/Main 1984.

Nathaus, Klaus: Organisierte Geselligkeit. Deutsche und britische Vereine im 19. und 20. Jahrhundert. Göttingen 2009.

Pfleiderer, Beatrix; Bichmann, Wolfgang: Krankheit und Kultur. Eine Einführung in die Ethnomedizin. Berlin 1985.

Pfleiderer, Beatrix; Greifeld, Katarina; Bichmann, Wolfgang: Ritual und Heilung. Eine Einführung in die Ethnomedizin. Berlin 1995.

Plagemann, Hermann: Der Wirksamkeitsnachweis nach dem Arzneimittelgesetz von 1976. Funktionen und Folgen eines unbestimmten Rechtsbegriffs. Baden-Baden 1979.

Regin, Cornelia: Selbsthilfe und Gesundheitspolitik: die Naturheilbewegung im Kaiserreich (1889 bis 1914). Stuttgart 1995.

Rothschuh, Karl Eduard: Konzepte der Medizin in Vergangenheit und Gegenwart. Stuttgart 1978.

Scheid, Volker: Chinese Medicine in Contemporary China. Durham 2002.

Stollberg, Gunnar: Volk und Gesundheit im Verein. Städtische Gesundheitsvereine von 1880 bis 1933. In: Reulecke, Jürgen; Gräfin zu Castell-Rüdenhausen, Adelheid (eds.): Stadt und Gesundheit. Stuttgart 1991, pp. 247–256.

Teich, Mikulás; Needham, Dorothy M.: A Documentary History of Biochemistry 1770–1940. Cranbury 1992.

Tsouyopoulos, Nelly: Asklepios und die Philosophen. Paradigmawechsel in der Medizin im 19. Jahrhundert. Ed. by Claudia Wiesemann, Barbara Bröker, and Sabine Rogge. Stuttgart-Bad Cannstatt 2008.

Medical Pluralism in Germany

Harald Walach

Introduction

In recent times it seems that "Evidence Based Medicine (EBM)" has become the panacea for all problems concerning medical regulations. During such times of inflationary usage of catchphrases it helps to go back to the roots and recall that the founding fathers of EBM had a triangulation of data sources in mind:

(i)   the best type of medical, scientific knowledge, stemming from research, ideally from randomised controlled trials and the synthesis of their results in a meta-analysis;
(ii) the clinical experience of the doctor;
(iii) the preference and wish of the patient as to how he would want to be treated.[1]

The reduction of the meaning of EBM to just scientific knowledge is not only short-sighted, preposterous and a sign of a lack of understanding, it is also dangerous. It is dangerous because it overemphasises perspectives that are by default limited in scope and directed at statistical ensembles, and thus neglects the individual perspective of patients. Hence it is not surprising that new initiatives, such as the German "Dialogforum" which tries to install a dialogue between conventional academic medicine and practitioners both in general practice and in complementary medical practice, are being started, that have as their goal the discussion of this plurality in treatment options, patients' wishes and choices, and the consequences for training and treatment.[2] This initiative is typically German, since it is in Germany that pluralism and various forms of complementary medical approaches, such as Hahnemann's homeopathy, Kneipp's naturopathy, Hueneke's neural therapy, treatments in medical spas and phytotherapeutic herbal treatments, have a long tradition. In this chapter I analyse this plural landscape in Germany, how it is presenting itself today, and what the political, societal and scientific consequences are.

Notions

Before we do that, let us clarify some notions. I have already introduced the term "complementary" medicine. This is often used to refer to non-standard

---

1   Sackett (1997).
2   Willich et al. (2004).

forms of treatments, not usually taught at medical schools but found in general practice, that are used to complement those standard treatments. In such an approach, non-standard treatments are used in conjunction with standard treatments. This is often the case if patients or doctors want to mitigate side-effects, support the system in general or treat aspects of a disease that cannot be treated conventionally. This terminology is often used in Germany and in Switzerland, where it has found its way even into the Swiss constitution.

If such non-standard treatments, such as homeopathy, nutritional approaches, usage of supplements or herbal remedies, are used in replacement of standard treatments, they are referred to as "alternative" medicine. Except in a minority of cases this is not the rule in Germany. For instance, in our own cohort study of a homeopathic treatment regime for cancer patients in a specialised clinic we saw that only 7.7% of patients in a homeopathic clinic and 1.1% of patients in a conventional cancer care centre declined conventionally indicated treatment and sought homeopathy as an alternative.[3] What is often feared and described in spectacular single cases – patients going for "alternatives" and neglecting necessary treatment – is not the rule, at least not in Germany and probably also not in other Western countries. It may, however, be the case for large parts of Africa and Asia.

Since the boundary between a complementary and an alternative usage of such non-standard treatments is rather fluid, the term "Complementary and Alternative Medicine (CAM)" was coined in the "Office of Alternative Medicine (OAM)" at the National Institutes of Health at the beginning of the 1990s. It is now a constituent of the "National Centre of Complementary and Alternative Medicine – NCCAM", the successor organisation of the OAM. It is widely used to designate this whole group of treatments which are not taught and researched as standard in conventional medical schools and hence are frequently not part of the public delivery system of medicine, often with the consequence that expenses have to be borne by patients privately. CAM is a term widely used, specifically in the US.

In the German discourse "Unconventional Medical Treatments" has been used, much to the same effect and for the same types of treatments. It is a more descriptive term in that it uses as a criterion of demarcation the fact that something is not part of the medical curriculum, whether or not it is used by patients in a complementary or alternative fashion. Although a descriptor in quite a few official documents – e.g. in a call for proposals by the ministry of research and various government reports – it seems a term out of favour with the public and is not often used.

What has become the leader of the hit list though, is the term "Integrative Medicine" or "Integrated Medicine (IM)". Pioneered by some American researchers, it has also captured the imagination of European authors. The catchphrase suggests that there is really only one medicine, not multiple ones and that whatever is empirically validated will eventually become part of this

3   Güthlin et al. (2010).

one medicine, no matter what its original background and model was. Thus, complementary approaches that are empirically supported will all become parts of the toolbox of a new, patient centred care with the goal of maximally serving the needs of patients and for the betterment of their suffering.

While this is a heroic stance that sounds very convincing and intuitive, I have raised some concerns in relation to it.[4] This is not because I think that the idea is not feasible. It is rather because I think such a stance is overly simplistic and overlooks an important aspect: Part of the reason why CAM has become so popular is due to the limitations of the current machine paradigm of the human being that is prevalent and endemic in current medicine and that treats the human body as complex machinery.[5] Patients intuitively feel that this model does not do justice to the complexity of their disease and its potential multiple causes and hence seek out a more holistic viewpoint.[6] Just integrating whatever fits the model of the current interpretation of EBM will also not do, because it might well be the case that some interventions will only show their full efficacy in certain contexts, and not in others. Hence, IM might just be a neo-colonialistic stance if used unwisely and without also considering, or rather reconsidering, the paradigmatic foundations of medical practice.

I refer to "Medical Pluralism (MP)" as a stance whereby various treatment options exist in parallel, are used by doctors and patients alike, and are allowed by the political system. The centrepiece of MP is the freedom of choice of doctors and patients, often seen as the freedom of the patient to choose a particular doctor or treatment and the freedom of the doctor to choose from various treatment options for the patient in question and to consider with the patient which type of treatment is most adequate for their problems.

During times when resources become scarce and Health Technology Assessment Agencies (HTAAs) try to define which treatment is good value for public reimbursement, such freedom sometimes becomes endangered and is sometimes dependent on the availability of private funds. While NICE, the National Institute for Clinical Excellence in the UK, the UK HTAA, regulates availability of choices, sometimes dramatically, this is not necessarily the case in Germany. However, another development is rapidly infringing on freedom of choice: the drafting of best practice guidelines in the wake of EBM. This reinforces the tendency of the medical profession to avoid law suits against malpractice claims and will rapidly limit pluralism simply because what is not referred to in guidelines as best practice will only be offered by doctors under severe caution, framed by indemnity letters which patients are required to sign.

It is quite telling to study the history of pluralism in Germany, a country which prides itself as the home not only of modern medical achievements but also of various other approaches, and to discuss its current state.

---

4   Walach (2010).
5   Walach (2011).
6   Furnham/Bhagrath (1993); Furnham (1992).

The History of Medical Pluralism in Modern Germany

The German statutory public reimbursement system is still in pretty much the same shape as it was when invented by Bismarck, the Reich's chancellor, in 1889. This is commonly considered the date when the current German social security system was put in place, and by and large the legislation can still be traced back to those days. The reason for this legislation has to be seen, of course, as so often in history, as the political attempts to make Prussia and the then united German nation an economically strong and powerful one. To achieve this, the country needed a system in which the ill were cared for and those in need of medical treatment would receive it. Hence a statutory insurance was introduced. Everyone who earned money paid into an insurance system out of which medical treatment was paid if someone was in need. Through rates that were in proportion to income everyone contributed to a similar degree and hence could take advantage of reimbursements.

Not only medical care was thus instituted for everyone, but also pension funds and funds to provide the rehabilitation of severely ill patients who could not be cured by a hospital stay alone. This is the basis of Germany's strong and unique rehabilitation sector. This is paid for out of public pension funds, and certain patients who have serious medical conditions due to a chronic disease such as asthma, depression, anxiety, rheumatoid arthritis, long standing back pain, chronic fatigue or other psychological or psychosomatic disorders, cancer, neurological problems, myocardial infarction and the like, can be given a prescription for a rehabilitation treatment by their doctor. This is evaluated individually and if found convincing by a panel of the rehabilitation sector the patient receives a defined rehabilitation treatment of three to six weeks, as a rule.

Rehabilitation clinics are entities that can offer their own individual treatment plans and normally cater for a particular set of diagnoses. They use a multi-pragmatic approach, often combining conventional treatments with complementary approaches and psychological or psychosomatic insights. Since patients have some choice, a market situation exists whereby successful treatment plans and combinations are sought out and thus reinforced by the system, while others are in danger of becoming unviable and hence abandoned. Rehabilitation clinics in Germany are, thus, a good driver for pluralism in the system.

The German statutory system is financed in part by employees who pay part of their salary into the health insurance, and in part by employers who pay another part into the system as an employee fringe benefit. Recently attempts have been made to introduce market mechanisms.

Insurance companies who have been part of the statutory system, as opposed to private insurers who can be used by freelance and self-employed persons or those with a high enough income, were able to introduce incentives, provide certain benefits such as free trainings or prevention classes. This has partially led to competition between such public insurers.

Also, hospitals and rehabilitation clinics have often switched ownership from public to private in recent years. While nearly all hospitals and rehabilitation clinics were either in public ownership – belonging to cities, towns, regional authorities and their legal entities – or owned by the churches, charitable trusts, or pension funds, privatisation has seen a takeover of many hospitals into private ownership, thus making them profit centres. Where ownership is still public, recent developments such as rising costs and scarcity of funds have reinforced a market mentality of making profit out of disease in what has been termed an illness economy.

Another element typical of Germany is the introduction of legal approval for a lay practitioner, the *Heilpraktiker*, in 1939 by the Nazi-regime. *Heilpraktiker* form a second strand of medical providers outside of the reimbursement system. They are typically paid out of pocket. Public statutory insurers do not pay for visits to them, although they may reimburse some of the medications they prescribe, but private insurers normally do pay for *Heilpraktiker* visits. Nevertheless they are still very popular in Germany, and their number is growing; in 2009 there were 30,000 *Heilpraktiker*, while in 2010 there were already 32,000.[7] Lay healer movements have always been strong in Germany.[8] Thus, consequentially, through an amalgam of tradition, lobbying, the need for a good medical provision for a whole nation on the brink of war and the Nazi-ideology of a new German healing culture (*Neue Deutsche Heilkunde*[9]), a new type of popular healer was introduced as *Heilpraktiker* into the German system. These people only had to prove that they have minimal knowledge so as to not be a health hazard to the population. Otherwise it was up to them how they gained their knowledge. Collaboration with doctors was legally prohibited. They were regulated by regional health authorities. These regional authorities used to have, and still have, some leeway in interpreting the legal framework and a wide variety exists in the way they implement the practice of examinations to fulfil the legal requirements. These lay healers played a strong role, being a competition with the mainstream medical model as well as providing the backdrop for patient choice and pluralism. While in the GDR the *Heilpraktiker* had nearly died out, probably due to a lack of political will to support a parallel system that was difficult to control, in the Western part of Germany and again in the reunited nation *Heilpraktiker* thrived due to a series of benevolent legal interpretations, passings of judgment, and clarifications of the opaque law. This allows persons trained in various therapeutic subdisciplines that are normally reckoned to be part of unconventional, non-mainstream practices, such as osteopathy or chiropractic, to become *Heilpraktiker* if they have the respective training. This will, in the long run and quite inevitably, lead to an academisation of certain traditions and a strengthening of plu-

---

7   Statistisches Bundesamt Deutschland, Gesundheitspersonal: https://www.destatis.de/
     DE/ZahlenFakten/GesellschaftStaat/Gesundheit/Gesundheitspersonal/Tabellen/Berufe.
     html (accessed 13 Dec. 2012).
8   Jütte (1996).
9   Rabe (1937); Rabe (1938).

ralism via this route of additional provision. It is easy to understand the political reasoning behind it: here we have a system of medical practice that is almost completely outside the statutory system, paid for and supported by patients, thus relieving the public system of burden and costs while at the same
time providing a strong backbone to the health economy.

The Current Situation

This development has led to the current state of affairs in which the system has
various strands:

1) The public statutory reimbursement system and a private insurance sector
   for the better off, financed by wages, compulsory for everyone and paying
   for all major health costs, especially for outpatient visits to GPs and specialists;
2) The hospital or secondary sector, financed by the statutory system and
   catering for all inpatient treatments, largely out of public funds but also
   supported by a manifold private insurance system that pays for extras and
   special treatment;
3) The tertiary or rehabilitation sector, financed by pension funds and funding specialised treatment for chronically ill patients;
4) A parallel system of lay practitioners (*Heilpraktiker*) that have freedom of
   treatment within their legal limits, but are not financed by the public reimbursement scheme.

This situation has led to a support of pluralism. By tradition, Germany has
seen a lot of medical movements, some of which have been inaugurated by
Germans, such as homeopathy, naturopathy, phytotherapy or anthroposophic
medicine and various mixed approaches. This situation has been paid tribute
to by legislation. Both in the German law on drugs (*Arzneimittelgesetz* [AMG]
§109a) and on the social system (*Sozialgesetzbuch* [SGB] V, §§ 34, 92) "unconventional" medical treatments are mentioned and specifically supported by
the law. The law states that homeopathy, anthroposophy and phytomedicine
are "special therapeutic disciplines" (*Besondere Therapierichtungen*) that need
separate legal provision. Thus, for example, in the regulation of drugs, separate conditions rule the process. For instance, homeopathic, anthroposophic
and phytotherapeutic drugs have to obey the same quality standards as conventional drugs. Appropriate fingerprinting and safety data are required,
whereby sometimes traditional usage criteria are enough. But efficacy data
need not necessarily be available if the traditional literature supports certain
usages. A simpler "registration" procedure allows the marketing of such drugs
which can be produced and sold in pharmacies for the usage of practitioners
and patients, without, however, giving indications. If indications are stated,

there needs to be a clearer support by the literature and, frequently, also additional clinical trials or observational data.

Thus, the German law caters for these specific therapeutic traditions and also acknowledges that there might be different standards of evidence due to their different tradition and usage. This general stance has, at least in general terms, been introduced into the European legislatory and regulatory framework. It does not affect already extant practices as in Germany, and allows countries that do not have such regulations to form new ones within the framework of a comparatively liberal legislation. There are limits, though, in that this regulatory framework is specifically geared towards supporting European traditions. Thus, homeopathy and anthroposophy is reflected, as is traditional European herbal medicine. This was, traditionally, a therapy that was rather fixed on single herbs or mixtures of few components, and hence the European legislation limits the amount of ingredients to six. This is not sufficient for Asian traditions, where multi-component remedies are the rule, but it supports the European traditions.

Social security legislation also caters for unconventional approaches. It allows public insurers to enter into so called test-phases. During such phases insurers can offer contested and new options of treatment or diagnostics to their patients under special conditions for a limited period of time, provided they have the delivery and its effects scientifically evaluated. This was used by insurers recently to propagate acupuncture and homeopathy through a series of studies.[10] While homeopathy can be offered by physicians in Germany who have the necessary qualifications and who work under the public system, acupuncture could not. This initiated the large German trial phase studies of acupuncture which became well known and were the reason for the introduction of acupuncture into the German system.[11] Thus, theoretically speaking, if an insurance company is interested in a new type of treatment they can offer it to their patients under regulated terms if accompanied by a scientific evaluation during such a testphase.

Problems with Pluralism

While this sounds all very nice, in practice the situation is less favourable. Here are a few examples: Homeopathic physicians are popular in Germany, as is homeopathy.[12] The German Association of Homeopathic Doctors has some 4,000 members, up from 2,037 in 1992[13], out of 439,090 doctors in total[14], i.e. roughly 1% of all doctors in Germany are officially homeopathic

10 Güthlin/Lange/Walach (2004).
11 Diener et al. (2006); Scharf et al. (2006); Haake et al. (2007).
12 Institut für Demoskopie Allensbach (2009).
13 Schüppel/Schlich (1994).
14 http://www.bundesaerztekammer.de/page.asp?his=0.3.9237.9238 (accessed 13 Dec. 2012).

doctors and have the title "homeopathic physician" which is regulated and provided by the regional medical boards. Even more doctors in Germany have taken the respective trainings. A lot of them work privately, but many also in the public system. They then get the same amount of money as do their conventional counterparts for a consultation. Through the limitation of the health budget what happens is the following: each and every doctor gets a certain amount, capped per patient and quarter. This amount is subject to negotiation and varies from quarter to quarter and also between geographical regions and types of practice, but is, roughly speaking currently between 30 and 70 Euros per quarter per patient. Thus, no matter what the doctor does, how much time he spends on a patient, he will always receive the set amount only. This forces doctors to see as many patients as they can per quarter, preferably only once in three months, in order to receive a decent income. Time, the prime resource of unconventional doctors, is not really reimbursed and hence unconventional practitioners tend to not work within the public system, and if they do, can only operate their skills to a limited degree. This produces the well known turnaround time of a German patient of roughly 5 minutes and is one of the reasons why a lot of patients seek out more "holistic" care in the private sector or with *Heilpraktiker*. The generic problem which the renaissance of complementary approaches seems to be an answer to is the lack of time and the fact that the way our system is currently organised does not support health but administers sickness. The German health or sickness sector is the biggest economy in the country, more important than the car industry or any other national industry. Many people profit from the fact that patients remain patients and do not become healthy. Economically speaking the best patient is one who needs medication on a continuous basis and is still able to work, who seeks out treatments but still lives long enough to pay the pension and insurance funds. Currently, it serves the purposes of the insurance companies if patients become diagnosed with more serious diseases, because they then receive additional funds from a state fund specifically created for that. An enormous overregulation that is the result of more complex guidelines and legal frameworks produces high additional costs for insurers who need to employ controllers and supervisors. This system limits the therapeutic potential of doctors in a general sense and reinforces dissatisfaction in patients.

Drivers for Pluralism

Patients in turn seek out other forms of treatments, more often than not in the private sector where most of the unconventional medicine can be found. Thus patients and their need for holistic treatment which is rarely supported by the public system because of the organisational restraints are the main drivers for pluralism. What they need and want cannot always be provided by the public system. The public system is diversified into specialist doctors, reflecting the great diversification of knowledge medical developments have generated.

While in other countries the science and training of general practice or family practice has been at the forefront, in Germany medical faculties have traditionally neglected the subject. During the recent initiative for excellence in academia, medical faculties have focused their resources even more in order to bid for excellence in areas where most scientific honours can be gleaned. These are not general practice but basic research like microbiology, genetics, and biochemistry. This leads to de-emphasising of practical clinical skills. Medical training is reflecting this, with practical skills not ranking topmost. The patients sense this and demand holistic practice from their GPs and where they do not get it they go out and seek it.

Thus the current pluralism is a complex structure with part of it being historical, part driven by patient demand, and part produced by the failure of the medical system to cater holistically for patients. One also has to consider that, mainly, doctors are doctors because they want to help patients, and not because their chief motive is to make money. They often experience that what they learn in medical school is not enough and hence seek out further trainings, often going into additional training with complementary medical teachings and schools.

In a study we did some years ago for an insurance company where patients could seek out homeopathic or acupuncture care, we asked them what the reason for this choice was.[15] 75% of these patients had chronic problems and had already seen conventional practitioners to no avail, and 73% were seeking out alternatives because of the side-effects of the medications used. Thus, a complex mix of a perceived lack of efficacy, side effects and a fragmentation of care, and the wish for holistic treatment drives patients to reinforce pluralism through their seeking of alternative and complementary treatments.

Researchers are also not to be neglected here. While not a large majority, young researchers have started to work in the field of unconventional medicine, starting back in the early 1990s. This has produced scientific evidence, some impact and discussion, and finally also some infrastructure. Of note, there have been eight endowed chairs and professorships of unconventional medicine or research in CAM in Germany recently. None of them are paid for by the public system, governments or universities, but all are supported either by charitable trusts, by hospitals, or by manufacturers of unconventional medications. This is an important step on the way to solidifying this pluralism which hitherto has only had grassroots and is now gradually shooting up into the further realms of academia. Interestingly enough research in CAM and the public have been forging strong links, as the public and public media have been, until very recently, on friendly terms with each other due to the fact that CAM was a publicly supported movement. This is changing gradually.

15   Güthlin/Lange/Walach (2004).

The Campaign against CAM

Over the last few years the public press, especially the mainstream print media, have become increasingly critical of CAM, mostly under the heading that treatments without evidence are costing money needed elsewhere or that research and training of such treatments in universities is defying rationality.[16] It is difficult to say what actually triggered this. But it is easy to observe that this campaign is waxing and waning in tides that are temporally correlated with bad news for big pharma. The campaign against homeopathy started in the UK after NICE banned new anti-dementia medication.[17] The campaign grew louder as meta-analytic results were published that severely questioned the usage and efficacy of antidepressants[18], and so forth. It is very difficult to overlook the correlation, but it is equally difficult to find causal links. Reframed positively this would mean that pluralism has finally become mainstream, at least in Germany and perhaps in wider Europe.

20 years ago CAM was a fringe movement with a few maverick researchers ploughing their way through the academic mainstream against a lot of obstacles, some ridicule and with support from very few but far sighted senior academics. Today CAM is a major part of new academic movements everywhere. There are at least 20 specialised journals in existence, with a yearly international conference, supported by an international scientific society (www.iscmr.org), testifying to the international appeal of the field. There are academic centres and research groups. NCCAM in the US has an annual budget of 150 million US dollars to support research. While this is not much in relation to the amount of mainstream funding, it is still a substantial sum of money. Major publications in mainstream journals have attracted attention, and the field has grown into a serious player, albeit a small and not very powerful one. Hence, the tradition of pluralism which Germany was always known for has, to some degree, been made fruitful by the worldwide renaissance of CAM and now IM, which has been, if not driven, then certainly made fruitful by the German tradition.

It is to be expected that the next wave of economic focus in the health system will actually benefit a plural standpoint. Economic consequences of CAM are not well studied. Where they have been studied, however, CAM always has proved to be beneficial.[19] German insurers know that unconventional treatments are comparatively cost effective. In our large cohort study of roughly 5,000 acupuncture patients who we followed for several years[20], we could demonstrate that work-days lost were reduced and quality of life improved. Others have shown that acupuncture or mindfulness meditation are

---

16   Colquhoun (2007); Walach (2009).
17   NICE (2006); Lancet (2005).
18   Turner et al. (2008); Kirsch et al. (2008).
19   White/Ernst (2001); Andrews (2005); Pelletier et al. (2010); Access Economics (2010).
20   Güthlin/Lange/Walach (2004).

cost effective interventions, perhaps not short term, but certainly long term.[21] At the moment insurers in Germany have no real benefit if they work cost effectively. Once they do, it is to be expected that they will reinforce cost saving strategies. One such strategy could be to support CAM treatments, either for certain conditions or even as a holistic family medicine strategy. Just recently a small German insurer, BKK-Securvita, started a new family medicine model, whereby doctors who have special training in naturopathy can receive special reimbursement within a package of family care.[22] The data are not available as yet, but what little we know would make the initiation of a study of conservative holistic and CAM treatment versus the interventionist stance that is currently prevalent plausible. One does not have to be a visionary to see that the odds might be on the side of the CAM treatments, although it would be necessary to really have robust data, which we currently lack.

Considering these factors altogether one can see that insurers could soon become drivers for pluralism. If I could become a visionary just for three sentences, my prediction would be: The future will be pluralist. The era of pharmaceutical companies as the dominant forces on the medical market is coming to an end, since they lack innovative products and ideas. A general shift in thinking and culture will reinforce the choice and responsibility of patients and that will, inevitably, create more pluralism. Thus, pluralism is the future, as it was the beginning of medical practice, since monoculture is unnatural and unsustainable, not only in ecological contexts but also in medical affairs.

Bibliography

Access Economics: Cost Effectiveness of Complementary Medicine. Canberra 2010.

Andrews, Gavin J.: Addressing Efficiency: Economic Evaluation and the Agenda for Cam Researchers. In: Complementary Therapies in Clinical Practice 11 (2005), pp. 253–261.

Colquhoun, David: Science Degrees without the Science. In: Nature 446 (2007), pp. 373–374.

Diener, Hans-Christoph et al., for the GERAC Migraine Study Group: Efficacy of Acupuncture for the Prophylaxis of Migraine: A Multicentre Randomised Controlled Clinical Trial. In: Lancet Neurology 5 (2006), pp. 310–316.

Furnham, Adrian: "Why People Choose Complementary Medicine." In: Yearbook of Cross-Cultural Medicine and Psychotherapy (1992), pp. 165–196.

Furnham, Adrian; Bhagrath, Ravi: A Comparison of Health Beliefs and Behaviours of Clients of Orthodox and Complementary Medicine. In: British Journal of Clinical Psychology 32 (1993), pp. 237–246.

Furnham, Adrian: Explaining Health and Illness: Lay Perceptions on Current and Future Health, the Causes of Illness, and the Nature of Recovery. In: Social Science and Medicine 39 (1994), pp. 715–725.

Güthlin, Corina; Lange, Oliver; Walach, Harald: Measuring the Effects of Acupuncture and Homoeopathy in General Practice: An Uncontrolled Prospective Documentation Approach. In: BMC Public Health 4 (2004), no. 6.

---

21 Vickers et al. (2004); Witt et al.: Cost-Effectiveness (2008); Kuyken et al. (2008); Witt et al.: Acupuncture (2008).

22 Ellis Huber, former Head of BKK-Securvita, personal communication.

Güthlin, Corina et al.: Characteristics of Cancer Patients Using Homeopathy Compared with Those in Conventional Care: A Cross-Sectional Study. In: Annals of Oncology 21 (2010), pp. 1094–1099.

Haake, Michael et al.: German Acupuncture Trials (Gerac) for Chronic Low Back Pain: Randomized, Multicenter, Blinded, Parallel-Group Trial with 3 Groups. In: Archives of Internal Medicine 167 (2007), no. 17, pp. 1892–1898.

Institut für Demoskopie Allensbach: Homöopathische Arzneimittel in Deutschland: Verbreitet, benutzt und geschätzt. Allensbacher Berichte (2009), no. 14, available at http://www.ifd-allensbach.de/uploads/tx_reportsndocs/prd_0914.pdf (accessed 13 Dec. 2012).

Jütte, Robert: Geschichte der Alternativen Medizin. Von der Volksmedizin zu den unkonventionellen Therapien von heute. München 1996.

Kirsch, Irving et al.: Initial Severity and Antidepressant Benefits: A Meta-Analysis of Data Submitted to the Food and Drug Administration. In: PLoS Medicine 5 (2008), no. 2, p. e45.

Kuyken, Willem et al.: Mindfulness-Based Cognitive Therapy to Prevent Relapse in Recurrent Depression. In: Journal of Consulting & Clinical Psychology 76 (2008), pp. 966–978.

Lancet: The End of Homoeopathy. In: The Lancet 366 (2005), no. 9487, p. 690.

NICE: Dementia: Supporting People with Dementia and Their Carers in Health and Social Care. In: NICE Clinical Guidelines 42 (2006).

Pelletier, Kenneth R. et al.: Health and Medical Economics Applied to Integrative Medicine. In: Explore. The Journal of Science and Healing 6 (2010), pp. 86–99.

Rabe, Hanns: Auflösung der Reichsarbeitsgemeinschaft für eine Neue Deutsche Heilkunde. In: Deutsche Zeitschrift für Homöopathie 16 (1937), pp. 3–4.

Rabe, Hanns: Homöopathie als Volksgut und als Wissenschaft. In: Deutsche Zeitschrift für Homöopathie 17 (1938), pp. 367–373.

Sackett, David L.: Evidence Based Medicine: How to Practice and Teach EBM. New York 1997.

Scharf, Hanns-Peter et al.: Acupuncture and Knee Osteoarthritis. In: Annals of Internal Medicine 145 (2006), pp. 12–20.

Schüppel, Reinhart; Schlich, Thomas: Die Verbreitung der Homöopathie unter Ärzten in Deutschland. In: Forschende Komplementärmedizin 1 (1994), pp. 177–183.

Turner, Erick H. et al.: Selective Publication of Antidepressant Trials and Its Influence on Apparent Efficacy. In: New England Journal of Medicine 358 (2008), pp. 252–260.

Vickers, Andrew J. et al.: Acupuncture of Chronic Headache Disorders in Primary Care: Randomised Controlled Trial and Economic Analysis. In: Health Technology Assessment 8 (2004), no. 48, pp. 1–47.

Walach, Harald: The Campaign against CAM – a Reason to Be Proud. In: Journal of Holistic Health Care 6 (2009), no. 1, pp. 8–13.

Walach, Harald: Complementary? Alternative? Integrative? In: Forschende Komplementärmedizin 17 (2010), pp. 215–216.

Walach, Harald: Weg mit den Pillen! Selbstheilung oder Warum wir für unsere Gesundheit Verantwortung übernehmen müssen – Eine Streitschrift. München 2011.

White, Adrian R.; Ernst, Edzard: Economic Analysis of Complementary Medicine: A Systematic Review. In: Complementary Therapies in Medicine 8 (2001), pp. 111–118.

Willich, Stefan N. et al.: Schulmedizin und Komplementärmedizin: Verständnis und Zusammenarbeit müssen vertieft werden – Mit dem Dialogforum "Pluralismus in der Medizin" soll ein Diskurs auf gleicher Augenhöhe in Gang gesetzt werden. In: Deutsches Ärzteblatt 101 (2004), no. 19, pp. A1314–A1319.

Witt, Claudia M. et al.: Cost-Effectiveness of Acupuncture Treatment in Patients with Headache. In: Cephalalgia 28 (2008), no. 4, pp. 334–346.

Witt, Claudia M. et al.: Acupuncture in Patients with Dysmenorrhea: A Randomized Study on Clinical Effectiveness and Cost-Effectiveness in Usual Care. In: American Journal of Obstetrics and Gynecology 198 (2008), no. 2, pp. 166.e1–166.e8.

Medical Pluralism – The Italian Case

Elio Rossi

Introduction

According to the results of the multipurpose survey 2005 on "Non-Conventional Medicines (NCM) in Italy" performed and published by the Italian National Institute for Statistics (ISTAT), 13.6% of the Italian population (around 8 million) had used NCM in the past three years.[1] The typical Italian user of NCM is an adult between 35 and 44 years of age with post high school qualifications; two thirds are women and the most used NCM are homeopathy, chiropractic/osteopathy, acupuncture and herbal remedies.

Complementary medicine (CM) in Italy

In Italy today there are almost 2,000 MDs using acupuncture, more than 7,000 homeopaths, about 20,000 MDs with a homeopathic training and approximately 200 MDs who have completed the course on anthroposophy. We can assume that there are at least 20,000 Italian practitioners (physicians, dentists, veterinarians) prescribing homeopathic, including homotoxicological, and anthroposophic medicines.

In Italy, homeopathic medicines are found exclusively in the pharmacy and they are sold by most of them. In the year 2000, at least 7,000 pharmacies out of 16,000 (43%), had a section for homeopathic and/or herbal remedies. At the moment, we can assume that around 90% of the Italian pharmacies offer homeopathic and phytotherapeutic products. In addition there are more than 4,000 herbal shops (*erboristerie*) regulated by law since 1931.

National regulation of CM

Italy is the third European country after France and Germany in terms of the size of the homeopathic and anthroposophic medicinal products market.

Italian Government and Parliament have been urged to pass a national law regulating the practice of NCM. No such national law has yet been passed. Since 1986, the year when the law was first proposed (by M. P. Garavaglia) more than 100 draft bills about NCM regulation have been tabled without result.

On 18 May 2002, at Terni, the National Council of the Italian National Federation of Medical Doctors and Dentists Associations (FNOMCeO) issued the "Guidelines of the FNOMCeO on non-conventional medicines and

---

1   Istituto nazionale di statistica (2007).

practices".[2] They recognized nine NCMs: acupuncture, traditional Chinese medicine, ayurvedic medicine, homeopathy, anthroposophic medicine, homotoxicology, herbal medicine, chiropractic and osteopathy. These practices are considered exclusively under the professional responsibility of medical doctors and dentists and must be formally recognized medical practices.

CM education

In 2009, the "Guidelines for non-conventional medicine and practices education" were published by FNOMCeO.[3]

They are a proposal for an agreement at the State-Regions and Provinces Conference on the criteria for CM training (amount of hours for the basic course, number of years, program, professional qualification of the teachers, etc.) and following on from what was proposed by the Interregional group on Complementary Medicine of the Health Commission of the Permanent State-Regions and Provinces Conference in 2008.

Continuing Medical Education in general (conventional) medicine is obligatory for all medical doctors in Belgium, France, Italy, Latvia, Lithuania, Slovakia (monitored by the government) and in Austria, Bulgaria, Czech Republic, Germany, Hungary, Poland, Romania, Slovakia, Slovenia, Switzerland and the United Kingdom (monitored by the national medical associations/chambers/councils). In Italy, complementary medicine courses are generally CME (Continuing Medical Education)-accredited.

At this moment we can consider that there are, or there were until last year, "High specialization courses", or "Masters", or "Elective courses" included within the basic teaching programmes of quite a number of Italian Universities, such as Torino, Milan Statale and Milan Bicocca, Brescia, Bologna, Florence, Siena, Pisa, Rome, Chieti, Cosenza, Palermo.

Italian National and Regional (Federal) Healthcare System

The Constitutional Law no. 3 of 18 October 2001 has reformed most of the Title V of the Italian Constitution (concerning regions, provinces, municipalities), making a so-called "federal system of state". The rule of the State (Government, Ministry, etc.) is to fix the "fundamental principles" on different subjects (education, urbanistics, etc.) and also in healthcare. The rule of the Regions is to decide how to put in practice and organize the public healthcare system according to the political and social perspective of each region.

For all Italian citizens, the "essential level of assistance" is guaranteed; which means that every person has the right to have a minimum (essential) level of healthcare, in any hospital of any region in the country.

2   Guidelines of the FNOMCeO on non-conventional medicines and practices (2012).
3   Guidelines of the FNOMCeO for non-conventional medicine and practices education (2012).

In the Regional Healthcare Plans (*PSR*) of Lombardy, Emilia Romagna, Tuscany, Umbria, Campania, Valle d'Aosta and Lazio, there are chapters about or references to CM. The regions have instituted regional commissions and/or scientific committees and/or Regional Observatories and/or regional structures of references for CM such as Campania, Emilia Romagna, Lombardy, Tuscany, Lazio, Friuli Venezia Giulia and Bolzano Province. Valle d'Aosta, Lombardy, Emilia Romagna, Tuscany, Umbria and Campania have given funds to support research on efficacy and economy of CM.

Information campaigns on CM or informative material have been published by the Autonomous Province of Bolzano, by the Regions Emilia Romagna, Lombardy, Tuscany and Campania, and moreover the Province of Bolzano has also supported associations and schools of CM. Refresher courses on CM for medical doctors and paramedical staff have been provided by the Province of Bolzano, by the Region Friuli Venezia Giulia, Lombardy, Tuscany, Campania and Umbria, and a survey of public clinics that provide CM service in Italy has been conducted by Bolzano, Emilia Romagna, Umbria and Tuscany.

CM included in the Regional Essential Level of Assistance

The Government Act DPCM of 29 November 2001 excluded acupuncture, phytotherapy, homeopathy and other CM, from the National Essential Level of Assistance (LEA).

In spite of this decision, some regions, such as Tuscany, Umbria, Valle d'Aosta, partially Campania and, only for specific research projects, also Emilia Romagna, have included CM in their regional LEA.

Until March 2006, according to a survey carried out by some CM Associations, there were at least 150 public complementary medicine clinics for out-patients in more or less all Italian regions.

Complementary medicine in the public health system: the Tuscany experience

The experience of the Tuscany Region in the integration of complementary medicine in the regional health system is widely considered the most significant in Italy and may be a reference for others wishing to follow in its footsteps. The result was achieved thanks to a joint effort of local CM associations and operators, despite belonging to different schools of thought and cultural orientations, in collaboration with the Department of Health and groups of the Regional Council interested in including CM in public health services. This joint work was aided by the spontaneous spread of these therapies in the region and the leading role of the Tuscan population in this sector.

The Tuscany Region is now a laboratory for innovations in this field. The most common forms of alternative (or complementary) medicine utilized are acupuncture and traditional Chinese medicine, herbal medicine and, finally, homeopathy.

Diffusion of complementary medicine and homeopathy in Tuscany

To explore the knowledge and the practice of complementary medicine and bio-natural disciplines in the Tuscan population, a survey has been conducted by the Regional Health Agency (ARS) of the Tuscany Region.[4]

In the 2009 survey, a random sample of 1,523 people aged 18 and over were interviewed by telephone. Complementary medicine was used in the previous three years by 11.5% of respondents (acupuncture 3.6%, homeopathy 7.9% and herbal medicine 1.8%). The most frequent users were people aged over 30 years with a high level of education. Regular physical exercise or a vegetarian or macrobiotic diet were predictors of CM use. 23.4% of respondents use homeopathy for their children and 3.1% for their animals. Most users obtained benefit from CM.

Practitioners and pharmacists turned out to be more involved in informing or advising patients about CM. Nevertheless, the main source of information or advice was relatives or friends, or even personal initiatives.

Only 18.8% of Tuscan residents (34.5% if we consider only CM users) know that CM has been recognised and introduced into its list of essential assistance levels by Tuscany. Most users pay for these services, even if they use the national health service to obtain them.

Bio-natural disciplines were used by 6.5% of respondents. The most frequently used are yoga (2.3%) and shiatsu (2.3%). Their users are younger than users of CM. Users (70–80%) have shown to rate CM highly.

Also significant is the number of people who have turned to complementary medicine in the public sector: around 50% of users contact practitioners with the public framework of the Health Service or National Health Service (NHS) and then inform their family doctors.

This trend is also observed in the data relating to specialized outpatient surgery departments constantly provided with information from the Region. Such data evidence a steady increase in the number of citizens who are turning to conventional medicine in the public health sector.

A different user profile emerges from the comparison of the ARS and regional investigation data. In the former case the age range is 31/45 years, in the latter it is 60/74 years for women and 65/74 years for men. More "mature" users choose the public sector and in particular acupuncture – the most common therapy in this field for the treatment of painful diseases. There has also been a marked increase in the use of complementary medicine in paediatric patients (more than 25%), and in particular of homeopathy (23.4%), also in the public sector.

---

4   Da Frè/Voller (2010).

Opinion of Tuscany doctors about CM

A survey on the opinions of family doctors and paediatricians working in Tuscany concerning the use of CM was conducted by the Regional Health Agency in 2003. 2,228 doctors and paediatricians were interviewed (of approximately 3,500 in total), with 82% supplying answers:

- 15.2% practise CM;
- 57.8% recommend them to their own patients;
- 11% have specific training;
- 29.2% would like to have training in CM;
- 65.7% are in favour of CM teaching at the university;
- 23.7% have used non-conventional medicine to treat their own ailments, compared to an average of 20% of Tuscan citizens, according to the 2001 ISTAT survey.[5]

The healthcare programmes of the Region of Tuscany

The healthcare programmes of the Region of Tuscany have contained references to various types of non-conventional medicine since 1996, and all recent Regional Health Plans have included a chapter on non-conventional medicine which arguably represents the greatest degree of integration of such therapies in the public health care system achieved in Italy so far. The aim is to guarantee definitive integration into the Regional Health Service of the types of non-conventional medicine that are supported by a sufficient level of scientific evidence to allow them to be defined as forms of complementary medicine (acupuncture, herbal medicine, homeopathy and manual medicine).[6]

Preliminary activities

The Regional Health Plan 1996–98 contained some regulations for the evaluation of "alternative medicine" and an invitation to look at "all practices of natural medicine and promote a health culture based on the reduction of the consumption of pharmaceutical products".

The first discussions on this issue took place at the conference held in Florence in December 1997 and were sponsored by the Tuscany Region. The aim was to stimulate reflection on the institutional dissemination of CM and to provide a concrete response to this phenomenon. In particular, the event called for the definition of programmes to transform the opportunities provided by the 1996–98 Regional Health Plan into initiatives and activities. From 1997 to 1999, for the first time in Italy, the Tuscany Region launched decentralized cooperation projects to support the development of natural medicine and homeopathy in various countries.

5   Giannelli et al. (2004).
6   Rossi et al. (2008).

The Regional Health Plan 1999–2001, for the first time in Italy, dedicated a specific chapter to complementary and alternative medicine and how it can be integrated into the regional health system. A CM Regional Commission of experts from different disciplines was also established with the task of identifying the strategies to achieve the integration of these medicines, even in veterinary medicine. The Commission had to identify instruments for assessing the demand for CM in the region; identify the most significant activities; evaluate proposals for research and define, with the medical associations and universities, criteria for accrediting training and establishing a register of CM doctors, and provide citizens with information on services and availability.

Among its first initiatives, the Commission, along with the Regional Health Centre, produced a survey to assess demand for CM in the Tuscany region, identify activities in the region, scientific and legislative documentation, the presence of acupuncture services, Traditional Chinese Medicine (TCM), homeopathy and herbal medicine within regional health service facilities, support for training and refresher courses for those involved in the public health service, as well as the testing of complementary therapies within the public sector.

In 1999, the Tuscan Regional Council allocated a special fund to support the development of CM activities in the regional health service on the basis of projects submitted by interested local health centres. In the summer of 2001, a resolution was approved to support research in this area (no. 628), which allocated specific funds. This enabled public and private institutions and associations in Tuscany to submit research projects to verify the effectiveness of complementary therapies in specific illnesses in both humans and animals.

The Regional Health Plan 2002–2004 made it possible to initiate a phase of more comprehensive and structured inclusion of these forms of medicine in the regional health system. The plan also included guidelines for general medical doctors on the use of these medicines and guidelines for the training of practitioners, in collaboration with the Tuscan Medical Council. In contrast to national provisions, which excluded CM from essential health services, the region approved not only acupuncture services but also homeopathy and herbal medicine, if included in specific projects.

Educational and training activities

The process of incorporating complementary medicines in the regional health system was developed in cooperation with the Medical Association and the Universities of Tuscany, who have organized activities in this field.

The Faculty of Pharmacy of the University of Florence has set up a course in advanced Chinese Herbal Medicine, the Faculty of Medicine and Surgery a level-II Master's degree in "Acupuncture and Traditional Chinese Medicine" and a level-II Master course in "Clinical Herbalism", in collaboration with the University of Empoli.

In 2007, the Faculty of Pharmacy of the University of Pisa introduced a level-I Master's degree course in "Medicinal and aromatic plants: raw materials for the food, cosmetics, pharmaceutical and health industry".

The Faculty of Medicine of the University of Siena set up a Master's degree course in Integrative Medicine in 2009. The universities of Pisa and Florence offer degree courses in herbal techniques.

A master's degree course in Natural Medicine (herbal medicine, acupuncture and TCM, manual medicine) has been set up at the Faculty of Medicine in Florence, starting with the academic year 2011–2012.

Communication

To facilitate communication, non-conventional and complementary medicine has been given a specific place on the official website of the Tuscany Region (Health section). The site contains information on the activities of complementary and alternative medicine in the region, legislation and an updated list of public CM structures at regional and national levels. The address is: http://www.regione.toscana.it/cittadini/salute/medicine-complementari (accessed 14 May, 2013).

There is also a regional newsletter for complementary and non-conventional medicine, *MC Toscana* (directed by Mariella Di Stefano). The newsletter is produced by the Toscan network for integrative medicine and the ASL 2 (Azienda Sanitaria Locale 2 – Local Health Unit 2) homeopathy clinic of Lucca. 2,500 copies of the paper edition are printed while the electronic newsletter is sent to at least 5,000 practitioners. The newsletter is published on the above-named site and is now in its 5th edition and 9th year of publication.

To disseminate information on complementary medicine as uniformly as possible, the Tuscany Region started an information campaign in the autumn of 2005. Adverts were published in the major regional and national newspapers, 220 posters and 5,293 adverts were displayed, and 265 adverts were placed on public transport. The communication initiative was about homeopathy, acupuncture and herbal medicine. For each of these forms of medicine a distinctive pathology was indicated, selected on the basis of CM effectiveness in available international literature and its occurrence within the population.

The complementary medicine sector takes part in various exhibitions and in particular, since 2004, in the Trade Fair *"Terra Futura"*, an international conference on innovations for good practices that are environmentally and socially sustainable (Florence-Fortezza da Basso). Thus, the Department for Health aims to propose a sustainable model of health that includes prevention and the promotion of public health care.[7]

---

7   Terra Futura (2012).

Complementary medicine in Essential Healthcare Services

The Regional Health Plan for 2005–2007 aims to integrate CM with sufficient levels of scientific evidence in the regional health service. They include acupuncture, herbal medicine, homeopathy and manual medicine. These types of medicine have been introduced in regional essential levels of assistance (LEA), with official price lists having been established. The plan also intends to approve a regional law to regulate practice; the inclusion of CM representatives in regional health council working groups (CSR); the introduction of regional guidelines, when they are recognized as an effective replacement, on complementary or alternative therapy for specific conditions; the promotion of information about degree courses on health; the implementation of specific activities that ensure integration in the regional health system, with a yearly budget of 600,000 Euros for the three-year period.

Moreover, the Regional Law N. 40 on "Local Health Centre Reform", passed in 2006 by the Regional Health Council and the Regional Bioethics Committee, provides for the presence of a complementary medicine representative in all Tuscan Health Centres (2 per centre).

With Resolution no. 655 (20 June 2005) complementary medicines were included in the official regional price lists. This enables residents to receive specialist treatment in acupuncture, homeopathy, herbal medicine and manual therapy for a fee of 18.59 Euros. Access to treatment is direct (no need to be referred by the family doctor).[8]

Regional law regulating bio-natural disciplines

In 2005, a regional law was issued regulating the practice of "Bio-natural disciplines" (BND). The definition includes practices such as naturopathy, shiatsu, reflexology, Tuinà, prana therapy, which stimulate the natural resources of the individual and are aimed at well-being and at improving quality of life.

Bio-natural disciplines also aim to encourage each individual to take full and conscious responsibility for their lifestyle and stimulate the vital resources of the person that is seen as a whole and inseparable entity.

Having established these common features, every discipline uses its own original approach, techniques and tools which are coherent with the specific cultural model to which the discipline refers. BNDs choose not to interfere in the relationship between doctors and patients and do not use drugs of any kind, because it is outside the competence of the practitioners specializing in these disciplines.[9]

---

8   Rossi/Di Stefano (2012).
9   Regional Law of Tuscany (2005).

Regional law on complementary medicine

In spring 2007, the Tuscan Regional Council approved the Regional Law of Tuscany no. 9/2007, which regulates the practice and training of complementary medicine by medical doctors, pharmacists and veterinarians. The legislation stipulates that medical doctors, dentists, veterinarians and pharmacists associations are to draw up lists of professional experts in complementary medicine based on the requirements defined by the Regional Committee for training in complementary medicine, and to issue a specific certification.[10]

The Regional Committee, established by the Directorate General of the Health Department, is made up of representatives of professional associations, CM associations, Tuscan universities, heads of the regional CM centres and experts appointed by the Regional Health Council. Public or private non-university training centres can be accredited according to law no. 993 of 9 November 2009.

A regional agreement was approved and signed on 8 April 2008 between Tuscany Region and Regional Federation of the Order of Doctors and Dentists, the Regional Committee of pharmacists and the Regional Federation of Veterinary Practitioners.[11] It defines the training and accreditation of complementary medicine professionals and training institutions and provides lists of CM professionals who practise acupuncture, herbal medicine and homeopathy. Those wishing to register must have a certificate issued by accredited public or private training centres and must have completed a course of no less than 450 training hours and 100 hours of clinical practice, after having passed a theoretical and practical exam and presented a dissertation. Courses for medical doctors and veterinarians cannot last less than 3 years. Training courses for pharmacists require at least 100 hours of theory and practice, and a course of no less than 1 year.

Transitional provisions for professionals who initiated the practice of complementary medicine before the law was approved were set up by April 2011. In addition to the basic principles and clinical application of complementary medical techniques, courses must ensure the teaching of medical criteria based on evidence, the capacity to conduct clinical research, and knowledge of legislation and regulations on rights to information and informed consent.

So far, six private training Institutes (5 of homeopathy and 1 of acupuncture), have completed the supervised accreditation procedure and their proposals were approved by the Commission for Complementary Medicine education and were finally accredited by Tuscany Region.

10   Regional Law of Tuscany (2007).
11   Modalita' di esercizio (2007).

Complementary medicine in specialist out-patient units

In September 2006 the Tuscany Region Integrative Agreement on specialist care for out-patients, which also includes complementary medicine, was signed, filling a gap in national legislation.

The agreement provides for the treatment of out-patients also by doctors specializing in complementary medicine and includes plans to bring the contracts of complementary medicine doctors working in local health centres in line with the economical and regulatory framework provided by the national collective agreement.

Specialists must have a certificate issued by the provincial medical association proving successful completion of theoretical and practical training that demonstrates expertise in complementary disciplines (acupuncture, herbal medicine, and homeopathy).

This is the first attempt, in Italy, to establish a procedure to which health services must adhere in order to offer complementary medicine within the public health sector, after a proper evaluation of the doctors' professional experience.[12]

Tuscan Regional Reference Centres and Network of Integrative Medicine

Since 1996, 106 public services for Complementary Medicine have been opened in Tuscany. There are 53 services of acupuncture and TCM, 27 of homeopathy, 14 of herbal medicine and 18 of other non-conventional therapies (manual medicine, etc.).[13]

The Regional Resolution no. 1384 (December 2002) established the "Regional Reference Structure for Complementary Medicine", made up of three regional reference centres: the Acupuncture and Traditional Chinese Medicine Clinic "Fior di prugna" of Florence, Local Health Authority 10, which is also the Coordinating Centre For Complementary Medicine in the region; the Phytotherapy Clinic of S. Giuseppe Hospital, Empoli, the Local Health Authority 11, which now has been transferred to the Careggi Hospital in Florence, and the Homeopathic Clinic of Lucca, Campo di Marte Hospital, Local Health Authority 2.

The "Tuscan Network of Integrative Medicine" (RTMI) made up of the public CM clinics was also established in 2007. It is an organizational model aiming to ensure a unitary system, integration, quality of services, safety for patients, with the objectives of prevention, therapy and rehabilitation. In 2009 it was recognized as a "regional structure of clinical government", alongside the Tuscan Transplant Organization, the Institute of Tumours of Tuscany, the Regional Centre for Clinical Risk and the Regional Blood Centre.

Finally, the Hospital of Integrated Medicine "Petruccioli" at Pitigliano in the Tuscan province of Grosseto opened to the public in February 2011. Inte-

12   Agreement (2012).
13   Complementary Medicine public clinics (2012).

grated services are available to citizens according to a health project promoting the therapeutic combination of traditional and complementary medicine. Patients are free to choose whether or not to turn to the integrated health service, whether in hospital or in an out-patient clinic.

Number of visits to public centres (2006–2010)

The data about the health services in complementary medicine in the period 2006–2010 allowed a detailed study of the services in this field.

In 2010, a total of 29,918 complementary medicine visits were provided by the CM services.

The number had been 19,698 visits in 2006, 22,812 in 2007, 22,551 in 2008 and 23,455 in 2009. Homeopathic were 5,982 in 2010 and 2,556 in 2006; and 20,857 in the five years under consideration. The patients who have access to public complementary medicine services mostly belong to the medium-to-high age range, in particular the age ranges 60/64 years and 70/74 for women and 65/69 and 70/74 for men.

The percentage of paediatric patients is much lower, with a prevalence (not uniform in the different local health authorities) of males over females. In general female patients prevailed over male patients: in 2010 there were 21,582 female patients versus 8,378 male patients.

Complementary veterinary medicine services

There are numerous veterinarians who use CM for the care of pets and farm animals throughout the region. The Rita Zanchi Homeopathic Veterinary School of Cortona (Arezzo), founded by Dr Franco Del Francia (died in 2011), has been running for over 20 years. An acupuncture course for veterinarians is available at the School of Acupuncture in Florence (directed by Dr Franco Cracolici). The Faculty of Veterinary Medicine at the University of Pisa is running a homeopathy clinic (Dr Francesca Pisseri) and a similar service is offered at the ASL 11 Empoli (directed by Dr Paolo Rossetti).

In the detention centre on the island of Gorgona (Livorno), which carries out agricultural, aquaculture and breeding activities, a pilot project has been running for several years on the use of homeopathic therapies in the treatment of animals, under the responsibility of Dr Marco Verdone.[14]

Aims of the Regional Healthcare Plan

In July 2008 the Regional Council approved the Regional Health Plan 2008–11 based on the principles of integration, freedom of therapeutic choice for users, freedom of treatment for doctors, service quality, training, research, user security and a networked organizational model for the public activities of

14   Gorgona (2012).

complementary medicine. Development guidelines aim to firmly establish CM activities in all healthcare centres, set up complementary medicine clinics in all Tuscan ASLs (Integrated Complementary Medicine Centres) and strengthen the Tuscan network model.

The regional development plan aims to define the training and accreditation procedures for CM professionals and training schools, identify scientific literature and evaluate the application of complementary and alternative therapies in oncology in order to define diagnostic and therapeutic guidelines, highlighting the contribution made by CM treatment in pathologies for which there is clinical evidence and studies in international literature that evaluate effectiveness. It aims to provide high level professional CM training for doctors and medical staff and refresher courses for health workers, family doctors, paediatricians and veterinarians, including those in the private sector, in collaboration with accredited regional schools. It also aims at the development of health monitoring programmes on adverse health effects related to CM, of relations with the Regional Bioethics Committee, and dissemination of accurate public information about the potential and the limitations of complementary medicine.

Attention should be drawn to the use of CM in family health clinics and birthing centres to improve women's health, promote natural childbirth and breastfeeding, and treatment of neuro-vegetative menopausal disorders; in activities related to childhood, the aim is to sustain growth, prevent and treat eating disorders and related behaviour, and to reduce recurring infections of childhood.

Complementary medicine is taken into consideration to improve the quality of life of chronic patients, the elderly and cancer patients and the mental health of adults and children, to combat pain, and for terminally ill patients (collaboration with the palliative care sector and regional hospices is considered an area of CM integration), to identify integrated procedures for the treatment of particularly widespread diseases like allergies, and finally to define intercultural models to address the health problems of immigrants.

Research carried out in collaboration with universities and private associations is of great importance. In addition to the effectiveness of therapies, research is concerned with gender-specific health problems, social diseases and rehabilitation, also the monitoring of user satisfaction, side-effects, potential reduction in spending on pharmaceutical products and medical tests. The contribution of CM and NCM in changing lifestyles will also be assessed.[15]

Regional Projects for Training and Research

Regional projects have been realized or are underway in the regional framework of the Integrative Medicine Network and Regional Reference Structures for these problems:

---

15 Regional Health Plan 2008–2010 (2012).

A) Regional working group "Complementary Medicine in Oncology", Tuscan Institute of Tumours and Tuscan Network for Integrative Medicine

Due to the widespread use of Complementary Medicine in oncology, the Tuscan Network for Integrative Medicine has set up an ongoing course about:

- Analysis of scientific literature (2005–2009), evaluation of the clinical experiences of Complementary Medicine in Oncology, evaluation of the application of complementary therapies in the treatment of cancer, on the basis of efficacy trials found in the literature and in consolidated experience.
- Identification of Evidence-Based Medicine (EBM) efficacy trials regarding the use of CM in the treatment of cancer. The searches will be classified according to the scale of the National Guidelines Project (2009).
- Training of healthcare professionals involved in oncology-related patient support.
- Diffusion of the use of CM methods which have proved useful in oncology within the public health structures.
- Information diffusion on cost/benefits concerning the use of CM among cancer patients. As a result of these activities, a Clinic for Complementary Medicine and Nutrition, promoted by the Clinic for Homeopathy and the Oncological Division of USL 2 (Unità Sanitaria Locale 2), Lucca, was opened in the District of ASL 2, Lucca, in October 2010. The aim of this structure is to use complementary medicine and nutrition to reduce the side-effects of tumour treatment and to improve the quality of life of anti-cancer patients.

A herbal medicine Out-patient Department of Oncology offering the service of acupuncture treatment was set up at ASL 11 of Empoli, at the Hospice of "San Felice a Ema" in Florence in 2010. Acupuncture, homeopathy and herbal medicine are provided to the oncology patients of Pitigliano Hospital.

B) Regional Course "Clinical Risk and safeness of the patient in Complementary Medicine", organized by the Tuscan Network of Integrative Medicine and Regional Centre for the Management of Clinical Risk

The compulsory CME-accredited regional course for healthcare professionals in the sector was conducted in 2009 to assess and monitor the clinical risk in diagnostic-therapeutic procedures relative to applied Complementary Medicine in the public sector of Tuscany.

Principal objectives:

- To assess and manage clinical risk in order to prevent adverse reactions to complementary treatment.

–   To guarantee the safeness of patients examined in the public centers of
    complementary medicine.

The Proceedings of the course were published in Italian as a supplement to
MC Toscana.[16]

C) Complementary medicine supporting natural birth

The training course "Delivery with Energy" addressed to Tuscan midwives,
has provided information on the methods of TCM which can be useful in this
field (Tuina Chinese massage, auto-massage, moxibustion, plum blossom,
rapeseeds, stimulation of auricular zones and Qigong exercises for instructor
training).

On the basis of this experience, a second training course in traditional
Chinese medicine, homeopathy and herbal medicine was applied to midwives.

The aims of the course are to:

–   enhance women's resources;
–   promote actions of self-management and update healthcare professionals
    in the methods of CM.

Interregional Group for Complementary Medicine at the Health Board

The Healthcare Board of the Conference State-Regions (22 February 2007) set
up a Standing interregional technical Group on Complementary Medicine, on
the basis of a document put forward by the representatives of a group of regions and laid down in 2006.

The main themes faced were research and training control in Complementary Medicine.

The Interregional Standing Group has been reconstituted in the present
legislature and coordination has been re-assigned to the Tuscany Region (Responsible: Doctor Sonia Baccetti).[17]

The international connections

Activities of health cooperation of the Tuscany Region with Cuba, within the
framework of natural and conventional medicine, and in particular of homeopathic medicine, were launched in 1994. Projects for decentralized cooperation have been realized in Cuba, Senegal, Serbia and with the Saharawi population of Sahara, with the cooperation of local bodies, international institutions, associations and non-governmental organisations (NGOs).[18]

16   Di Stefano/Rossi/Bellandi (2010).
17   Rossi/Baccetti (2011).
18   Rossi et al. (2010).

An international Seminar "Innovation and Development in the Health System: inclusion of complementary and traditional medicine in the Public Health System", promoted by IDEASS, the program ART/UNDP Tuscany and Tuscany Region, was held in Florence in October 2008, with the participation of delegates and experts from Afghanistan, Albania, Austria, Bolivia, Chile, Cuba, Ecuador, El Salvador, France, Gabon, Germany, Guatemala, India, Iran, Italy, Lebanon, Mali, Morocco, Mozambique, Dominican Republic, Serbia, Syria, Sri Lanka, Switzerland, South Africa, Venezuela, the Agencies of the United Nations and bodies of international and decentralized cooperation.

The event ended with a declaration referring to a number of key factors on the subject of integration: the intercultural approach for health, respect of human rights, protection of natural resources, principles of complementarity, reciprocity, inclusion and respect for nature and the environment.[19]

Since February 2011, Tuscany Region (as Tuscan Network for Integrative Medicine and Tuscan Tumours Institute) has been an "associated partner" of the *"European Partnership for Action Against Cancer"*, initiated by the EU Commission in September 2009 with the support of a number of stakeholders such as the European Cancer Patient Coalition (ECPC), and bringing together the Commission, Member States and their Ministries of Health, patient organisations, health professionals, scientists, private industry and civil society. The region has embarked on an ambitious agenda of a pan-European collaborative effort to tackle cancer more evenly and effectively across the EU.

The task of Tuscany within the Work package no. 7 (WP7) is to assess the evidence and use of complementary medicine (CM) in cancer care and to propose criteria for the dissemination of appropriate information; assessment of dissemination of CM, review of the evidence and mapping of the EU CM in cancer care.[20]

The last step was the organization of the 5th European Congress of Integrative Medicine (ECIM) in 2012, which had taken place so far in Berlin and in Florence (Italy), and on 21–22 September 2012 the Congress, entitled "The Future of Comprehensive Patient Care Promoting health and developing integrated and sustainable treatment for acute and chronic diseases", was organised by Tuscany Region, General Directorate of Health Department, and by the Tuscan Network for Integrative Medicine, with the Charité University of Berlin, Institute for Social Medicine, Epidemiology, and Health Economics, in co-operation with the University of Florence, the other Tuscan Universities and the regional Chamber of Medical Doctors and Dentists (http://www.ecim-congress.org, accessed 14 Dec. 2012).

It was the main European and international event for physicians, healthcare professionals, scientists, and sponsors on the efficacy of complementary/non-conventional medicines and their integration with conventional medicine. The congress offered an innovative platform and promoted the exchange and positive dialogue of best medical practice.

19   International Workshop (2008).
20   European Partnership for Action Against Cancer (2012).

The aim of the Italian ECIM was to promote the exchange between medical doctors and researchers, and the dialogue and debate on experiences with the integration of complementary/non-conventional medicines in the National Health Services of Northern and Central Europe and those of Mediterranean countries.

ECIM 2012 also hosted the XXVI GIRI Congress (Groupe International de Recherche sur l'Infinitésimal), about the biologic effects of very low dose and ultra-diluted substances (http://www.giriweb.com/, accessed 14 Dec. 2012). This event was organised by Prof Paolo Bellavite (University of Verona) and Prof Lucietta Betti (University of Bologna). Many other events of domestic and international scientific societies were also held.

Conclusions

Tuscany's case is not isolated in Italy, even though the same levels of integration have not been achieved in other regions. Despite having contrasting outcomes, there are numerous regional initiatives of various types concerning training, complementary medicine services available to the general public and legislative initiatives.

Complementary and traditional medicine can represent a useful and sustainable resource in different fields of healthcare: chronic disease, lifestyle, natural childbirth, allergies, cancer, pre- and post-operative rehabilitation, epidemics, paediatrics, third age, dentistry, veterinary medicine. Their inclusion in the public health system must go hand in hand with an adequate process of scientific validation to control the efficacy, safety and quality of the health services and products by means of case/control observational studies, as well as randomized and double-blind clinical trials for the treatment of pathologies of particular social interest. Major initiatives and concrete actions aimed at achieving strategies of inclusion of complementary and traditional medicine in the public health care systems also regard the introduction of these disciplines in regional and national health care planning, in the programmes of public health structures, and the approval of specific regional and/or national norms. Particular attention should also be given to programmes for the training of public health care workers, for University graduate and post-graduate vocational training and ongoing professional refresher courses. Finally, information provided to the citizens is a question of primary importance for the development and success of integration courses.

Acknowledgements

We thank Dr Laura Cignoni for the English translation and Dr Mariella Di Stefano who contributed to the bibliographic research and revision of the text.

Bibliography

Agreement for the regional discipline of relations with medical specialists in hospital clinics, available at http://www.aupitoscana.it/wp-content/documents/convenzionati/accordi_regionali/accordo-regionale-2006.pdf (accessed 19 Dec. 2012).

Complementary Medicine public clinics of Tuscany Region, available at http://www.regione.toscana.it/regione/multimedia/RT/documents/2011/07/08/e5253dbef969b88c5d0e-a46b84bc5456_censimento2011tascabile.pdf (accessed 14 Dec. 2012).

Da Frè, Monica; Voller, Fabio: Regional survey on Complementary Medicine, Bio-natural and Wellness Practices (2010). Unit of Epidemiology, Regional Health Agency of Tuscany, available at http://www.ars.toscana.it/aree-dintervento/cure-e-assistenza/medicine-complementari.html (accessed 19 Dec. 2012).

Di Stefano, Mariella; Rossi, Elio; Bellandi, Tommaso: Sicurezza del paziente e gestione del rischio clinico in medicina complementare. In: Supplement to MC Toscana Bulletin no. 18 (2010), available at http://www.usl2.toscana.it/documenti/pubblicazionesicurezzapazienti-rischioclinico.pdf (accessed 19 Dec. 2012).

European Partnership for Action Against Cancer (EPAAC): http://www.epaac.eu/ (accessed 14 Dec. 2012).

Giannelli, Massimo et al.: Non-conventional medicine in Tuscany: attitudes and use in the population. In: Epidemiologia e prevenzione 28 (2004), no. 1, pp. 27–33.

Gorgona: similitudini in tracce, available at http://www.ondamica.it/?p=1306 (accessed 14 Dec. 2012).

Guidelines of the FNOMCeO for non-conventional medicine and practices education, available at http://www.omceomb.it/public/upload/Normativa/Linee_guida_FNOMCeO_formazione_nelle_medicine_e_pratiche_non_convenzionali.pdf (accessed 14 Dec. 2012).

Guidelines of the FNOMCeO on non-conventional medicines and practices, available at http://www.omceomb.it/public/upload/Normativa/Linee_guida_FNOMCeO_formazione_nelle_medicine_e_pratiche_non_convenzionali.pdf (accessed 14 Dec. 2012).

International Workshop "Innovation and development in health: Integration of complementary and traditional medicine in public health systems" 28–31 October 2008 Florence, Italy, Final declaration, available at http://www.universitasforum.org/index.php/ojs/article/view/71/267 (accessed 19 Dec. 2012).

Istituto nazionale di statistica (ISTAT) [National Institute for Statistics]: Le terapie non convenzionali in Italia [Non-conventional medicine in Italy]. Anno 2005. Roma 2007, available at http://www.istat.it/salastampa/comunicati/non_calendario/20070821_00/testointegrale.pdf (accessed 14 Dec. 2012).

Modalita' di esercizio delle medicine complementari da parte dei medici e odontoiatri, dei medici veterinari e dei farmacisti. Protocollo d'intesa (ex Legge Regionale n°9 del 19 febbraio 2007) [Practice of Complementary Medicine by Medical Doctors and Dentists, Veterinaries and Pharmacists. Memorandum of intent of R. L. n. 9/2007], available at http://www.regione.toscana.it/regione/multimedia/RT/documents/1207822728762_49_com.pdf (accessed 14 Dec. 2012).

Regional Health Plan 2008–2010 of Tuscany, available at http://www.regione.toscana.it/regione/multimedia/RT/documents/1216825956079_5_nuove_opportunita.pdf (accessed 19 Dec. 2012).

Regional Law of Tuscany no. 2/2005, Wellness and Bio-natural Disciplines, available at http://www.regione.toscana.it/regione/multimedia/RT/documents/2009/08/06/ea83ab7fc7d-c8915a59169bcbe0f3f74_legge22005.pdf (accessed 14 Dec. 2012).

Regional Law of Tuscany no. 9/2007, available at http://jtest.ittig.cnr.it/cocoon/regioneToscana/xhtml?doc=/db/nir/RegioneToscana/2007/urn_nir_regione.toscana_legge_2007-02-19n9&css=&datafine=20121214 (accessed 19 Dec. 2012).

Rossi, Elio et al.: Homeopathy and complementary medicine in Tuscany, Italy: integration in the public health system. In: Homeopathy 97 (2008), pp. 70–75.

Rossi, Elio et al.: International cooperation in support of homeopathy and complementary medicine in developing countries: the Tuscan experience. In: Homeopathy 99 (2010), pp. 278–283.

Rossi, Elio; Baccetti, Sonia: La pratica clinica delle MnC nell'ambito del SSR in Toscana. In: Proceedings of XI Convegno A.M.I.A.R. Agopuntura e Medicina Non Convenzionale: integrazione nella pratica clinica. Torino 2011, pp. 35–42.

Rossi, Elio; Di Stefano, Mariella: Complementary and alternative medicine in the health system of the Tuscany Region. Integration and innovation for health, available at http://www.regione.toscana.it/regione/multimedia/RT/documents/2009/07/22/5c3cc2b0b7c2ba100f8fd450c41722c5_brochuremedicinecomplementaritoscana.pdf (accessed 14 Dec. 2012)

Terra Futura: http://www.terrafutura.info/ (accessed 14 Dec. 2012).

Medical Pluralism in the UK – A Personal View

George Lewith

Introduction

This personal view is my experiential and iterative understanding of how medical pluralism, in particular the development of complementary and alternative medicine (CAM), has evolved in the United Kingdom over the last 30 years. It is history as it unfolded in response to the political and social changes that have occurred within this area.[1]

The enthusiasm of the 1980's

As the student expression of revolutionary change during the late 60's and early 70's began to wane an active and now employed minority of educated professionals began to perceive that there were perhaps other unconventional ways to approach the promotion of health and management of illness. A number of older physicians also began to reflect on their lifetime's work in medicine, realising the power and strength of the individual therapeutic relationship and how that formed an essential part of the physician's armoury[2] that was at the core of good medical practice. This enabled the establishment of a number of active pro-CAM groups firmly embedded within conventional medicine. The Research Council for Complementary Medicine was established in the early 1980's (http://www.rccm.org.uk, accessed 14 Dec. 2012) and groups such as the British Medical Acupuncture Society began training GPs to offer acupuncture as part of normal clinical practice (http://www.medical-acupuncture.co.uk, accessed 14 Dec. 2012). The British Holistic Medical Association (BHMA) was also established with much fanfare and created an approach that saw general practice offering a broad range of NHS funded therapeutic interventions with its home base in the Marylebone Church Crypt (http://www.bhma.org, accessed 14 Dec. 2012). This was achieved with very limited opposition and much support from the conventional medical profession. The BMA was initially trenchant in its view that these approaches were unacceptable but subsequently its later policy and strategy made it very clear that it wished to work with GPs and CAM practitioners interested in complementary medicine, facilitating a process of improved dialogue and increasing professionalization for CAM.

1   Sharma (1992).
2   Lewith (1987).

A series of Royal Society of Medicine colloquia entitled "Talking Health" formed an important and dynamic focus for discussing these issues[3], and many senior physicians were happy to contribute in an open, thoughtful and constructive way laying the groundwork for future professionalization of CAM and indeed the development of thoughtful and focused research environments in which these therapeutic interventions could be scientifically investigated.

The expansion of the 1990's

During the 1980's and 1990's one almost had the feeling that the media at large were uncritically positive of CAM. It was as if the "alternative counter culture" of the 60's had somehow become accepted by the establishment; Saks talks about this social and political evolution in a neo-Weberian context. The UK government enabled general practitioners to hold their own budgets and approximately 40% of GP surgeries spent this on offering some kind of primary care CAM service, often including acupuncture and osteopathy for the management of musculoskeletal pain.[4] The Prince of Wales's Foundation for Integrated Health took a lead in the development of these issues and brought together the British Medical Association and the Royal Colleges (primarily the physicians and general practitioners) and was a driving force behind the discussions that enabled research support through Department of Health Capacity Building Research awards scheme. The open development of doctoral and post-doctoral research fellowships led to a small but significant expansion in interest and research capacity within the UK. Our research output, clinical practice and investment in this area was second to none in the UK.

The House of Lords' Report

The House of Lords' Report was a very thorough investigation of the state of complementary medicine, clinically, professionally and academically. It laid vital groundwork for the structure and development of CAM.[5] The Prince's Foundation for Integrated Health took on the role of managing the regulatory process and very rapidly osteopaths and chiropractors became statutorily regulated. A similar process involving acupuncturists and herbalists has evolved over the last decade and the result is that herbalists are now regulated and acupuncturists are not. The Complementary and Natural Healthcare Council was established (http://www.cnhc.org.uk, accessed 14 Dec. 2012) with the help of the Foundation and the Department of Health helping to manage and regulate the voluntary sector (areas such as aromatherapy or reflexology and heal-

3   Watt/Wood (1988).
4   Thomas/Coleman (2004).
5   Saks (2003).

ing). Slowly but surely CAM in the UK has divided itself into those who wished to become "statutorily regulated practitioners, equivalent to doctors, nurses and physiotherapists" and those who wished to remain in the voluntary regulated sector offering a complementary medical approach that supplemented conventional medicine. In some therapies, such as homeopathy, the long UK tradition of medically qualified and medically regulated homeopaths remained as well as an increasing number of non-medically qualified voluntarily regulated homeopaths represented by organisations such as the Society of Homeopaths.

Opposition emerges

As the Department of Health capacity building research fellowships came on stream, a number of academics began, apparently, to see this as a threat to their research funding and credibility. Opposition began to emerge from surprising quarters, including amongst those who felt aggrieved that they had been completely unable to obtain peer review research funding within this field and the battle lines began to be drawn. Anything that seemed to be remotely connected with complementary medicine was deemed as semi-religious and unscientific whereas the religion of evidence-based medicine (scientism) was seen as acceptable science in spite of its self-evident academic and scientific inadequacies when applied to the vast majority of medical consultations in primary care. The recent initiative created by the Obama administration to develop comparative effectiveness research (http://tiih.org/about/team.php, accessed 14 Dec. 2012) is based on the fact that current medical research in the Western industrialised nations was failing to provide the evidence required by physicians faced by increasingly complex clinical issues.[6] The evidence that was available is often expensively obtained and inappropriate.

One of the great achievements of the National Institute for Health Research in the UK has been to create a coherent and clinically focused research agenda which has largely moved away from the placebo controlled trial to evaluating patient preference and safety and cost-effectiveness of the interventions available to clinicians as the basis for logical, thoughtful, safe and constructive clinical decision making by the National Institute of Clinical Excellence (NICE).

However, within the context of the media there is little doubt that during the last decade the main UK broadsheets and the majority of the scientific press have substantially changed their view in relation to CAM becoming as irrationally anti CAM as it was previously irrationally supportive during the 1980's. We are now in a position that almost whatever evidence is produced the media and scientific establishment (including some of the major medical

6   Sox/Greenfield (2009).

journals) report this inadequately and perceive the data to be poor and inadequate science promoted by incompetent and uncritical individuals.

The role of the NHS and the provision of CAM

The UK has one main provider, evaluator and purchaser of healthcare. The NHS is the largest employer in Europe and is fundamentally conflicted in terms of its many functions. Largely because the NHS is politically driven and embedded in our culture, it has a policy to provide high quality healthcare to all those in need, irrelevant of their means.

At the same time, the financial constraints imposed by increasing medical technology and the limited economic capacity to pay, create huge conflicts between management and clinical professionals, as well as between various government departments about the relevant political and social priorities that the UK should pursue. Furthermore, UK patients have, in effect, very limited choice about which doctors they can see and the doctors themselves are increasingly guided and directed as to what they can provide for whom. There is therefore a very limited capacity for patients to either seek complementary medicine through the NHS or indeed for the doctors to provide it. This has in effect meant that the majority of CAM provision within the UK has been within the private sector.

Cancer is an interesting case study in this context. The UK appears to be largely unable to offer an integrated cancer health service within the constraints of the NHS as the private sector is able to offer in the United States, but is more than happy to offer a superbly integrated palliative care environment through which almost all the CAM interventions are made available to those with terminal disease. Cancer services are research based within the NHS and driven by randomised controlled trials as well as being exclusively doctor dominated. Palliative care is a charitable partnership between the NHS and largely patient driven with an emphasis on improving the quality of life and death for both the patient and their family. Somehow our approach to this area is beautifully encapsulated in the very different ways that these two medical environments are funded and prioritised and consequently how and to whom they are able to deliver a pluralistic and responsive model of care.

Conclusion

The UK was one of the first Western industrialised nations after the Second World War to begin to think about how it may be able to offer and regulate a truly pluralistic medical environment. The growth of rational discussion and clinical services on offer in the UK during the 1980's and 1990's created real consumer choice irrelevant of ability to pay. The political and economic backlash that has occurred over the last decade has seen these developments eroded. Most worryingly, the excellent academic foundations laid down during the 1990's are now deteriorating so we may never really have the strong, thoughtful and self-critical academic institutions through which the evidence-based pluralism demanded by patients might have evolved.

The use of complementary medicine by the population has not diminished in the UK, quite the reverse; there are indications that it is slowly but surely increasing and now approximately 15–20% of the UK use or purchase some form of complementary medicine each year. The institutional response to this has been to fly in the face of the public will and marginalise CAM in terms of NHS healthcare provision. Not only does it appear that the UK wishes to marginalise CAM practice, it also seems not to want to know anything about how these interventions might be impacting on patients' health, well-being and self-care. CAM faces a period of political marginalisation in which for now the culture of medical scientism and the misguided but apparently dominant belief that we really do have an evidence-based treatment for our chronic long-term conditions appears to hold sway.

Bibliography

Lewith, George T.: Every doctor a walking placebo? In: Complementary Medical Research 2 (1987), pp. 10–17.

Saks, Mike: Orthodox and Alternative Medicine: Politics, Professionalization and Health Care. London 2003.

Sharma, Ursula: Complementary Medicine Today. Practitioners and Patients. London; New York 1992.

Sox, Harold; Greenfield, Sheldon: Comparative effectiveness research: a report from the Institute of Medicine. In: Annals of Internal Medicine 151 (2009), pp. 203–205.

Thomas, Kate; Coleman, Pat: Use of complementary or alternative medicine in a general population in Great Britain. Results from the National Omnibus survey. In: Journal of Public Health 26 (2004), no. 2, pp. 152–157.

Watt, James; Wood, Clive (eds.): Talking Health: Common concepts in conventional and complementary medicine. London; New York 1988.

Medical Pluralism in Health Care –
Experience from New Delhi

R. K. Manchanda and Harleen Kaur

Introduction

With the world witnessing a revolution in the way biomedicine is perceived in this 21st century, the room for discussion and deliberation on the way the human body is understood by the complementary therapies has widened like never before. Medical science is transforming at a fast pace, and the novel ideas are surprisingly bringing 'modern' science closer to the 'traditional' one – with ideas of holistic treatment and life space investigation becoming not only acceptable but imitable, as conventional medicine rethinks its perspective towards human health and objectives behind case interrogation. The paper explores various dimensions of medical pluralism in India and mulls over the new adaptations that India needs to make to sustain the present growth and emerge as a global player in the field of homeopathy.

Evolution of Medical Pluralism in India

India has been a country of interest for the medical historians, with its history of medicine dating back to the primitive era, with *'Charak Samhita'* and *'Sushruta Samhita'* documented in about 1000 B.C. Ayurveda, the ancient Indian medicine, originated long back, with some scriptures like *'Rigveda' and 'Atharvaveda'* being 5,000 years old. The tradition of Yoga was also born in India several thousand years ago. Its legendary founders were great saints and sages. The *'Siddha'* system is another one of the oldest systems of medicine in India, with its origin in the south of India. Even today it is practised largely in the Tamil-speaking part of India. However, India has long remained under the rule of a foreign dynasty, and with the changing kingdoms, the country came under the influence of the varied treatment methods practised by the ruling kingdoms of the respective period. This saw the advent of the *'Unani'* system of medicine in India from the 13th century onwards, first with the establishment of Muslim rule over North India and subsequently flourishing under the Mughal Empire.[1]

In the mid-19th century, the colonization of India by the British brought the western systems of medicine to India.[2] Since homeopathy had many adherents in a number of European countries during that period, a few Chris-

---

1   Cf. Bagchi (1997).
2   See Poldas (2010), especially pp. 17–38.

tian missionaries, who settled by the side of the River Ganges in West Bengal, introduced this system of medicine to a few Bengali physicians. Dr Johann M. Honigberger (1795–1869) is a name that comes up prominently in this context. He is credited with having introduced homeopathy in India in the 1830s. The concept of the 'immaterial or dynamic essence' was in harmony with the traditional Indian values that instilled in one the belief in 'what was beyond the domain of seeing, or feeling or touching'; or in other words, what was immaterial. While allopathy had made deep inroads in the country till then as the 'Angrezi' (British) medicine, the homeopathic system struck the right chord in the Indian minds for bearing a unique combination of being 'western' and still not away from the Indian core beliefs about the human body and human existence. Thus homeopathy flourished in India. The first homeopathic hospital was opened in India as early as 1852 in Calcutta. Since then homeopathy has gained considerable momentum in India which is now a 'superpower' in this field of therapy.

Institutionalization of Homeopathy in India

Realizing its growing popularity and acceptance in the public, in April 1937, Md. Ghias-ud-idin, a member of the Central Legislative Assembly (CLA) of Punjab, moved a resolution for the recognition of homeopathy. The resolution was passed and forwarded to the State Governments for its implementation. Bengal was the first province to constitute a Homeopathic State Faculty in 1943.

The Homeopathy Central Council Act, to provide for the constitution of a Central Council of Homeopathy and maintenance of a Central Register of Homeopathy and for matters connected therewith, was passed in 1973. Understanding the need for further research studies in this relatively new system, the Government of India planned to establish the Central Council for Research in Homeopathy (CCRH), an autonomous research organization, in 1978.[3] The policies of the government of India have been encouraging and supportive of promotion of homeopathy. Homeopathic doctors enjoy the same status as allopathic doctors in a government dispensary and draw an equivalent salary. To further promote homeopathy, more and more medical colleges have been opened by the Central Council of Homeopathy, with the current total being 186. The introduction of a post-graduate course, M.D. (Hom.), has provided further thrust to the cause of spreading homeopathy in this country.

This clearly reveals that as regards governance and various policies, homeopathy is enjoying a comfortable position in this country. If one adds to that the large number of homeopathic medical colleges and the even larger number of homeopathic followers among the masses, India will any day be a

3   Official website of Central Council of Homoeopathy: http://www.cchindia.com (last accessed 14 Dec. 2012).

paradise for homeopaths. This wide acceptance, both by the public and the government, is the reason why homeopathy has reached the level where it is today in India.

Experiences from New Delhi

A few surveys done by the Delhi Government about homeopathic practice in comparison to allopathic practice revealed interesting facts:[4]

- Expenditure in homeopathic clinics was one-fifth of that in allopathic clinics, both in terms of salary and medicines.
- The morbidity profile of both types of clinics revealed that diseases of the respiratory tract, infections, gastro-intestinal (GIT) diseases and skin diseases are the most common diseases at Primary Health Care (PHC) level. The patterns showed that patients were not similar in allopathic and homeopathic clinics. These clinics complemented each other. Allopathic treatment was found to be preferred by patients with acute diseases and homeopathy by those with sub-acute and chronic diseases. This preference indicates the strengths and limitations of these systems, in the perception of the public.
- The majority of the doctors of allopathic clinics felt that homeopathic clinics within the same premises are beneficial for the patients.
- The doctors expressed that they do not face any problems in running both clinics and also refer the patients to homeopathic clinics for treatment.
- The awareness among 383 (45%) patients was through word of mouth (patient to patient contact). This indicates the acceptability of homeopathy among the general population.
- The patients attending homeopathic clinics were from various occupations and all strata of the society.
- The patient satisfaction levels were very high and gratifying. Only 1% of the patients were dissatisfied with homeopathic services.
- Of all the patients surveyed, 85.2% felt that the homeopathic system of medicine is better than other systems of medicine. The study showed that patients also visited the allopathic clinics and other clinics depending on their requirements and preferred to use different systems of medicine according to their experience and advice of physicians.
- Most of the patients were of the opinion that homeopathy was safe, easy to take, cost effective and had faith in homeopathy due to their past experiences.
- The surveys concluded that homeopathy is a popular, affordable and efficacious system of medicine at primary health care level and bears the potential to minimize health care expenditure substantially if promoted in

4   Manchanda/Kulhashreshtha (2005).

primary health care through the 'cafeteria approach' adopted by the Government of Delhi.

Adaptation of Health practitioners to society needs

However, introspectively, this acceptance of 'one and all' itself is very 'Indian' in nature. Medical pluralism has never been contentious in India. It exists at various levels. At patient level, a typical Indian patient is never wary of choosing from available treatment options. Especially, the word-of-mouth appreciation works like nothing else in an Indian family. People tend to believe that what has worked for him shall work for me too. At the government level, both the state and central governments have not yet been able to balance the demand and supply curve in medical care, especially in the rural areas. The governments aim to incorporate trained medical practitioners of various systems of medicine in the health services, in order to meet the ever-increasing health demands of the Indian population. Furthermore, this medical pluralism very much exists at the physician level too. A physician of one science doesn't seem to refrain from prescribing medicine from the other science. It is not uncommon to see an allopathic physician prescribing an ayurvedic or a homeopathic medicine, or an ayurvedic or homeopathic doctor prescribing an allopathic medicine. The latter group, in fact, exists in a large number, especially in the rural areas, where the medical aid is too narrow and the range of illnesses too wide. A homeopathic physician practising in a remote village of India might confide to prescribing allopathic medicines, or even conducting minor surgeries, for that is the kind of demand in the villages. And to his mind, not all the illnesses of rural people can be treated homeopathically – blame it on the lack of time per patient owing to long queues, or on the lack of faith of the villagers in anything that is not in tablet or capsule form. But in a broader perspective, this group of homeopathic doctors only improvises to meet the needs of that section of society, and it might not be that easy to blame them for the service they are providing, sitting there in a remote village. Urban homeopaths, in contrast, are more homeopathy-oriented and faithful to their system. Besides, within the cult of homeopathic doctors there is pluralism too. Of late, many schools of thought, with varying approaches to treating patients, have emerged. All these schools promote homeopathy, but the analyzing and prescribing techniques vary from one another. The one may call himself a classical homeopath and prescribe only single remedies in single doses, while the other may prescribe only on the basis of mental make up of the patient. Then there are schools that focus more on the physical constitution and still others who prescribe self-formulated or patented combinations of various medicines. By practising in this way, they still promote homeopathy and benefit the patients, besides bringing renown and a good reputation to homeopathy as a whole.

India – Growing in isolation?

On the flip side though, despite such huge support and widespread acceptance, Indian homeopaths have not been able to put the available opportunities to the best advantage. When it comes to standardized, evidence-based research or well-documented cases, India still needs to go a long way, and perhaps learn from its smaller but more informed counterparts of the western
world. India has the largest homeopathic infrastructure in terms of manpower,
institutions and drug manufacturing industry, which can be effectively utilized
globally. To achieve this, Indian homeopathic education needs the right orientation to attain finesse in clinical acumen. The physicians need to focus on
reaching the diagnosis of every case being treated with homeopathy; prescribe
on definitive indications of drugs so that, on the basis of clinical experience,
earlier data can be validated; start treatment with low potencies 3x, 3, 6, 12
and then go higher as required in each case; give adequate doses of drugs to
ensure cure and treat cases to logical end and stop running after miracles.
Similarly, the drug industries need to be more focused on quality assurance
regarding their pharmaceutical products. Lastly, our homeopathic community
should be willing to join hands with mainstream medicine in areas where the
scope of homeopathy is limited or known to be merely palliative.

Conclusion

We have seen that medical pluralism or the 'cafeteria approach' exists in the
very 'system' of India. Given these attributes, it has been a triumphant task for
the homeopathic leaders of India to bring homeopathy at a par with other
systems in the government, of course, not without their share of struggle and
persistence. However, for the counterparts in the other parts of the world, a
replication of the Indian model of success might be a tougher call. However,
India, knowingly or unknowingly, has become a clear case in point as to how
and what can be done to make homeopathy an integral part of primary health
care services in other parts of the world too. With the available statistics and
huge following, India is today the second home of homeopathy. Can there be
more similar homes for homeopathy? It is for all of us to contemplate.

Bibliography

Bagchi, Asoke K.: Medicine in medieval India: 11th to 18th centuries. Delhi 1997.
Manchanda, R. K.; Kulhashreshtha, Mukul: Cost effectiveness and efficacy of Homoeopathy
    in Primary Health Care Units of Government of Delhi – A study presented in 60th World
    Homoeopathic Congress at Berlin, Germany, from 3rd May to 8th May 2005 organized by
    LIGA Medicorum Homeopathica Internationalis, available at http://www.homeo.delhig-
    ovt.nic.in (last accessed 14 Dec. 2012).

Poldas, Samuel Vijaya Bhaskar: Geschichte der Homöopathie in Indien. Von ihrer Einführung bis zur ersten offiziellen Anerkennung 1937. Stuttgart 2010.

Medical Pluralism – Past and Present: Towards a more precise concept

Martin Dinges

Introduction

In this collection of essays important aspects of medical pluralism in Europe, past and present, are addressed by various authors. This contribution is not a summary of the various contributions but a reflection on some of the key issues. A central question is the historical development of medical pluralism: one may ask whether it makes sense to apply this term to such widely differing moments in history as the years 1600, 1800, 1900 and 2000. No doubt the medical market of skills and services was already quite different in 1800 from what it had been in 1600. One just needs to consider the vanishing role of religious healing and the "decline of magic", that had taken place in the interval. The change was even more obvious 100 years later, when the discoveries of bacteriology had established the new paradigm of scientificity as a constitutive element of "modern" medicine – rather narrowly self-defined by the clinicians and understood by the larger public as a "science based on research". Efficacious therapies followed much later – the antibiotics, which were only made widely available in Europe after World War II, were certainly another landmark. To get a more precise picture of the historical development it seems appropriate to look for *thresholds* which mark important steps in this development.

Various points in time have recently been proposed in this respect. The one most discussed has been the distinction between "old" and "new medical pluralism" (Cant/Sharma), which highlights the contemporary changes since the end of the assumed predominance or "monopolistic" position of the biomedical paradigm from the 1980s onwards and fits in best with the striving to understand the modern world as it is.[1] From a more systematic point of view, one could derive a third phase from this model: the time before the establishment of "modern" biomedicine. But the centuries preceding the twentieth are largely ignored in this conceptualization. The dichotomy of "old" and "new" is not really satisfactory for the historian – and the lack of interest in earlier centuries even less.

To cover these remote times Stollberg, in his contribution to this volume, distinguishes between medical *plurality* and *pluralism*, the crucial difference being that plurality is a social field with a variety of healthcare providers and a diversity of medical systems, medications and therapies without much competition for scientific or professional supremacy as neither science nor profes-

---

1   Cf. introduction to this volume; for homeopathy see Dinges (2012).

sions in the modern, sociological sense exist. Pluralism however includes an "active engagement with diversity or plurality", in our case a political bargaining between providers and their "medical systems" and an (implicit or explicit) theoretical reference which is common.[2] That might be a reference theory such as biomedicine, it might also simply be the idea of medicine as science. I shall take up his suggestion below.

Another sort of definition of medical pluralism underlines the character of medicine as culture. This approach is intended to avoid the rigidities of the term "system". Traditionally, systems are conceptualized with clear-cut boundaries and relatively stable interior relations between their elements that produce a certain structure. The problem is that medical systems rarely meet these requirements because they tend to be more fluid.

Medical cultures as reference?

Medical cultures – as a specific set of meanings – might at first sight be better suited to the purpose of analyzing medical plurality or pluralism. The existence of at least two different medical cultures and the encounter and interactions between them was and is the norm in history. Europe, for instance, inherited much from Graeco-Roman tradition which was to a large extent transmitted and modified by the Arabs. In medieval Europe a medical tradition was constantly being created by integrating various local experiences and older elements into an emerging corpus of medical knowledge which also had intimate links with magic and religious healing. This is certainly a good example of medical plurality. I would not use the term "medical pluralism" for this epoch. There were no clear-cut borders between "learned medicine", "popular medicine" or the "medicine of the other" in a sense of Arab medicine or medicine from outside Europe.

This state of affairs seems to have changed very slowly, beginning with the European sea-faring expansion, commonly dated from 1492 onwards. With the discovery of the Americas and the Indian Orient, consciousness definitely emerges of the different medical heritage of the "New World" – with many new substances entering Europe as a result.[3] Later, during the 17th century, an attempt was made by physicians to draw a sharper line between certain non-Christian religious and magic healing practices outside Europe and parts of the christianized population inside this continent – but this did not much affect the practice of other healthcare providers (cf. Ramsey in this volume) or even the physicians themselves, who share many elements of their materia medica with "popular medicine". The conscious internal differentiation of the medical knowledge mainly concerns the elite – the new substances were integrated into practice – to a large extent by the official care providers – as was the case with Guajak and the treatment of syphilis as early as the 16th centu-

2   Cf. Jütte (1998), pp. 66–69.
3   Cook (2007).

ry.[4] One must doubt whether this could already be named "medical pluralism". It seems much more an example of a successful appropriation of new
substances and their integration into practice through the medical establishment – but not yet a dialogue or even a political bargaining with "the other"
based on theory. It enlarges the plurality of the medical field.

Status of healthcare providers crucial?

As the reference to knowledge or to "foreign" substances fit for medical usage
does not lead to a precise criterion for defining a threshold as a starting point
of medical pluralism, focusing on the healthcare providers seems a better approach. From the moment when two or more healthcare providers deliver
different medical services there is an element of medical plurality. This was
certainly the case as long as there were religious and magic healers and various medical healers such as physicians, barber-surgeons and lay practitioners.
The pharmacists, who always tended to give advice and to practise medicine
were another group which had been separated, at least theoretically, from the
physicians since the statutes of Frederic II of Sicily 1231/40. But it took until
the 17th century for these regulations to be implemented – even in Soest, which
was a large German town in the late Middle Ages.[5] As long as these providers acted in a complementary way without much declared competition and
did not base their treatment on distinctive bodies of knowledge, a consciousness of "medical pluralism" in the sense of an "active engagement with diversity" could not emerge. It was just a medical market that offered a variety of
providers, medications and practices. As Ramsey demonstrates in his contribution to the French example, until late in the 16th century it was still possible
to discuss what "being a physician" or "doctoring" actually meant. The dividing lines between the various "health-professions" were, for a long time, not as
clear as we might expect if we consider the terms "medicus" or "physicus" and
the legal framework. It seems to me that another element must be added – the
establishment of a hegemonic position of one group of healthcare providers –
so that a more relevant prerequisite for medical pluralism can be established.

Physicians claimed quite early on that they were the most competent specialists for diagnosis and have had legal confirmation of this claim since
1231/40. But they did not necessarily claim to be the best specialists for all
sorts of treatments. Up to well into the 19th century they preferred to have
most surgeries carried out by the barber-surgeons. It was also not until the first
third of the 19th century that physicians began to act as a kind of backup in
more difficult cases of childbirth, an area that until then had been almost entirely left to the midwives.[6] But physicians had already claimed a right to
control the admission to the "office" of midwives in German imperial towns

---

4   Stein (2003).
5   Jankrift (2003), p. 47.
6   Schlumbohm (2012); Seidel (1998).

during the late 15th century.[7] Town physicians were also obliged to control the pharmacists. The autonomous barber-surgeons had long been independent artisans with a professional training, but the limits of their field of activity – only external treatments – had been clearly defined by physicians since the late Middle Ages. And, as Jütte emphasizes in his contribution, it was also the physicians who had declared the outbreak of an epidemic since late medieval times. These examples illustrate the idea of a "hegemonic position" of physicians: to a certain degree the physicians tried to define the space for the other medical professions, without necessarily considering them as competitors.

As a result the town physicians played a growing role in public health, especially concerning epidemics – after the plague and until the Late Enlightenment (1350–1750/70); and in another very limited field we see very slow growth with regard to formal rights to oversee further aspects of the training or practice of minor medical "professions" where public health was concerned. But efforts towards implementation in city-states and territories remained weak. As a result the (English) medical market of the 18th century could still be characterised by R. Porter as a time of "low therapeutic efficacy, a high degree of pluralism, a high degree of consumer choice and lay participation, and the rise of a new market-based medical consumerism" (Nicholls).

It is the final step from hegemony to domination which makes the difference. Physicians defining themselves as exclusively competent was certainly not a sufficient prerequisite for such dominance: it needed legal confirmation and an institution powerful enough to impose the new rules of medical dominance. The period beginning with the last third of the 18th century seems to me crucial: physicians were establishing themselves definitely as the specialists, advising the rulers on all sorts of problems concerning public health such as hygiene, childbirth, the training of midwives, dietetics, population growth, hospitals, epidemics, pharmacies, the quality of water and its supply, a healthy environment, cemeteries, military medicine and many other fields – not forgetting the personal health of the ruler. And the legislators tended to increasingly confirm the pivotal role of physicians in the medical realm. From the early 19th century onwards, the hospital as the locus of clinical research, training of physicians and – as the third priority – treatment of patients has been instrumental in fortifying the ever more hegemonic and ultimately dominant role of the physicians, which was largely achieved before World War I – in terms of public recognition and legal and economic status. As Bauberot shows in his paper, in France the cooperation of the state with the physicians to implement their prerogative remained minimal even beyond the middle of the 19th century.

---

7   Flügge (1998).

Bodies of knowledge

Therefore medical pluralism seems to me a useful term for medical markets where, firstly, one group of providers that offered distinctive medical services not only rejects other bodies of knowledge but claims a dominant position for its own ideas – in our case biomedicine as defined by science as a theory of reference (Ernst) or a reflective theory as Stollberg terms it in this volume – and, secondly, this dominance is socially and legally recognized. In a situation where one group of providers claims and/or maintains only a hegemonic position, I would prefer to use the term *"medical plurality"*, because the market is less competitive and the hegemony has less exclusive effects. It is not really implemented politically. The crucial difference to medical pluralism is that no dominant position of biomedicine in terms of importance, funds and general recognition has been achieved yet, as was the case in the later long-term European, if not global, development. It is the pretention of exclusiveness and its power-based implementation which creates modern medical pluralism (cf. Bauberot).

Advantages and disadvantages of a narrow concept of medical pluralism

This concept of medical pluralism is deliberately defined in a particularly narrow way as it is based on the reference to a certain body of knowledge and the group of providers. This seems to be an advantage: with this definition not every medical market on which various medicines and treatments circulate at any time in history and in any place on the globe represents "medical pluralism". Such an understanding of medical pluralism seems to me heuristically not sufficiently clear cut to support useful scientific distinctions. The definition of physicians as dominant providers also makes it clear that this type of medical pluralism is based on a very specific idea of medicine: it is neither health, nor the patient, nor the treatment that are at the centre of this concept of medical pluralism, but a specific group of providers with a specific theory of reference – biomedicine – and the legal background of a state. This does not even exclude the possibility that a fraction of these biomedically trained physicians refers in their practice to other theories such as homeopathy – as long as the prerequisite of the status of physician is not called into question. This seems at least the position of the European Union and the German legal framework.[8] It might be seen as a form of medical pluralism in which CAM is domesticated under biomedical dominance. At the same time this arrangement might indicate the limits to dominance.

---

8   The German "Heilpraktiker" – a certified lay practitioner, who has passed an exam under supervision of physicians and has limited allowances for treatment except e.g. contagious diseases – is the exception in European law.

Medicine as a healing practice or as an art, as an interaction between an ill person and a physician or lay practitioner is not in the foreground. All the crucial points of a debate on health and healthcare provision are relegated to a secondary role. This must be kept in mind when using the term "medical pluralism" in this narrowly-defined sense. This implies that the hierarchical structures of the market are first considered. Therefore power and inequalities between providers inside this stratified market become a central issue of research. Access to resources such as money from the patient – or later from insurances and national healthcare schemes –, access to training institutions such as universities and to the patient become crucial.[9]

Such a market in itself has a profound effect on the health education of the patient, on his ideas regarding the importance of dietetics and lifestyle, his responsibility in matters of health, the imagined role of health-care providers, the pattern of use of health-care institutions and, ultimately, the efficiency of healthcare as such. It also shapes the interaction between an ill person and the treating person.

Other definitions of medical pluralism are possible but I fear that they do not distinguish sufficiently between plurality and pluralism and are therefore less useful. One may nevertheless ask whether it makes sense to introduce a term like "old medical pluralism" (1900/20–1980) or even "medical proto-pluralism" (1780–1900/20). This concept could serve to distinguish various steps on the way towards full-fledged modern medical pluralism. An argument in favour of such a proposition could be that it would allow a better differentiation of the centuries since 1231/40 by following the various changes after the Black Death, the age of discovery or during Late Enlightenment. On the other hand it might suggest a teleological view of history: as if all earlier times were only the preparation or preliminary stages of modern times – which is a frequent implication when conceptualizing history as a process of modernization. This trap should be avoided. But it might be useful to distinguish various phases of medical plurality. As explained above, the changes in the impact of physicians in all health affairs were very gradual from 1231/40 until 1900/20 and one may ask whether such a distinction would be at all useful. This seems even more the case if one considers the eminent contribution of lay practitioners and other non-academically trained healers to healthcare throughout European history – even if it is difficult to establish their market share in quantitative terms.

Triggers of historical change: bringing the patient back in (to medical pluralism)

It seems to me heuristically more enlightening to think about changes in the last 30 years. Considering the physicians and their dominant body of knowl-

---

9   It is up to further discussion what it really means that under the British poor law any kind of profession was employed but no physician.

edge in our definition as crucial for the establishment of medical pluralism, leaves the important question open as to the role the patients played in this development. Demanding all sorts of treatment that might promise to improve their health, patients were always an important driving force for plurality inside the medical market – from antiquity to the present. The concept of the commodification of medicine implies that medicine has changed since the 18th century and become a commodity – something people may buy like any other service or product.

The idea is that with the beginning of the consumer society – from this quite early point in time, at least for the upper classes – the character of the interaction between medicine, physicians and the patient began to change in a fundamental way. We may leave the discussion about the roots of our society aside, but refer to it in order to ask whether the trend towards further differentiation – and one might say more medical diversity – has not had a new quality since the 1980s. Is the patients' demand nowadays a significant driving force inside the established medical pluralism towards a more diversified market?

It is quite evident that the public took a critical stance towards the two pillars of the established system: firstly, biomedicine as a reference "theory" which seemed to exclude holistic forms of healing when applied to therapies.[10] Among other factors, as early as the 1960s the scandal involving a tranquilizer (Thalidomide) which, after consumption by pregnant women, led to the birth of deformed babies, interfered with the shining image of biomedicine.

The second pillar was the role of the physician as the sole and only authority of health, to whom the patient would have to submit.[11] A critical minority asked for change in the interaction between patient and physician towards more equality. Seeing the physician as the exclusive specialist became less and less accepted. He even triggered a much more general criticism of specialists in modern societies. This was underscored by the observation that biomedicine was not the solution for every health problem as physicians, surgeons and the pharmaceutical companies had stylized it during the last two decades leading up to 1980. More and more chronic diseases subsisted in an ageing society with ever elder patients despite impressive medical, pharmaceutical or surgical achievements and successes. This was certainly more a problem of communication than a real failure of the medical system: the medical system fell short of the inflated expectations it had generated.

In any case, patients articulated their needs not only individually or inside families but also in various forms of social movements – as women, homosexuals, AIDS-sufferers and in many other self-help associations – which were finally able to emerge as a political lobby. As Marland shows in this volume, already in the 19th century patients' guidebooks could contribute to dissemination of ideas of medical plurality. From the 1980s, critical patients at last found

10   Capra (1983); Illich (1977); cf. Dinges (1996).
11   Dinges: Aufstieg (2013).

a larger audience in the media which could become a driving force for the advancement of knowledge about CAM and its wider use.

In my opinion it was less the long-term development towards the commodification of medicine that made the difference: the national insurance system in Germany dates from the 1880s, the one in France from the late 1940s, as does the NHS in the UK. Even before 1900 patients, if and when they were represented in the administration of such systems, sometimes facilitated the introduction of CAM inside these schemes. But these were exceptions. In general, these quite monolithic national systems did little towards creating a wider space for CAM inside the system.[12] In Germany the competing private insurance companies discovered CAM in the 1990s as an inducement to attract new subscribers and, in some rare cases, they even funded research (Walach).[13] Around the turn of the millennium some insurance companies discovered that they wanted to find out more about the cost and benefit of CAM in general. This led to some of the most interesting studies on the use of CAM in Europe. For the Netherlands and Switzerland, such solid studies involving large numbers of patients provided evidence that competent CAM-physicians were able to treat patients more cost-effectively on the long-term than their colleagues without CAM-knowledge.[14] Under the particular conditions of the Swiss democracy with its high level of participation the patients as voting citizens were able to force the health authorities to assess the potential benefit of including CAM into the statutory healthcare provision via a neutral national institution. The result was positive in terms of "clinical and preclinical efficacy" and led to the reintroduction of funding such therapies by the national insurance scheme.

On the other hand, the British National Council for Science and Technology, which evaluates government policies in this field criticised the lack of scientific proof – for example of homeopathy. Interestingly, the British government nevertheless refused to stop funding this form of complementary medicine by the NHS. The crucial argument was the free choice of the patient and the confidence in the competence of the physicians.[15]

This shows that the use of CAM has become so politicised, that exclusively clinical arguments – with their very particular understanding of efficiency – are no longer sufficient for political decision-making on the national level with regard to the place of CAM in medical pluralism. The political standing of CAM may vary from country to country, with the current official attitude being positive in Germany and Italy, reticent in Poland and the UK, which had promoted CAM inside medical pluralism in the 1970s (Nicholls).[16] But wherever the patients have more influence on the public debate, CAM has better chances to play an important role. In conclusion I suggest that the

---

12 A short-lived exception is Germany after 1933, cf. Bothe (1991); Alfred Haug (1985); Roswitha Haug (2009).
13 Kooreman/Baars (2012).
14 Kooreman/Baars (2012); Studer/Busato (2010).
15 Cf. Dinges (2012).
16 Walach/Weidenhammer (2012).

"new medical pluralism" has led to certain changes in the health policies since the 1980s: during the last generation patients were more successful in making themselves heard and had more impact on the choices inside an established medical pluralism that does question the pivotal role of the physician.

At the same time the image of the patient has changed. He is no longer the heroic figure or association member who fights for his or her emancipation against the medical specialist but the consumer of commodified medical services, concerned about the side effects of invasive therapies and ready to try new ways and means such as CAM. Considerate doctors responded to this demand and extended their services to include CAM. This flexibility of the medical system allowed the physician to maintain his central position – under slightly changed conditions: a bit more informed consent and a bit more CAM.

Perspectives

1) The subject of this volume, medical plurality and medical pluralism, was initially construed by ethno-medicine and anthropology as being located "outside of Europe". As a consequence it has too often been seen as a strange phenomenon, belonging more to "the colonies" than to Europe. The contributions to this volume invite reconsideration of these assumptions, that still seem to prevail – at least outside the academic disciplines of anthropology and ethnography – for example in parts of the history of sciences or in general history. Medical plurality is and was much more of a constant element of European medical history than it might have seemed during the short period of the biomedical "monopoly" that lasted from the 1920s to the 1980s and covered two generations. The term "hegemony" seems more appropriate for the role biomedicine played during that period, since it underlines the central position of biomedicine. Its standards of scientificity were the crucial point of reference of all other medical systems but biomedicine never attained a monopolistic control of the market. The medical market in Europe remained much more pluralistic than the dominance of biomedicine in the faculties and in the public debate might have suggested since 1950.[17]

2) This volume concerns mainly medical plurality and medical pluralism in Europe, more precisely in some of its larger countries, principally Italy, Germany, the United Kingdom and France. It is not impossible that at least the chronological development which we tried to establish might be different if we included the countries of the Balkans and Eastern Europe into this comparison. The later and weaker bureaucratisation especially in the eastern parts of the continent leaves a much larger margin for all sorts of non-academically trained providers over a longer period of time. Additionally, the magico-religious medical market is different in the realm of the orthodox church than in catholic or even protestant countries.[18] One may ask to what extent these

17 Mildenberger (2011).
18 Cf. the reference Gentilcore makes in this volume to Papadopoulos.

denominational backgrounds, which later often transformed into specific national scientific cultures, played a role in the continued existence of medical alternatives. The strictly administrated Lutheran countries of Scandinavia, for example, have kept a greater distance to all forms of complementary medicine, from when the image of biomedicine as "scientific" was established during the 19th century to this day.[19] This certainly did not convince all members of society: Danish patients knew as well as French patients how to get hold of the CAM medicines for self-medication that were forbidden in their countries – not yet via internet but by mail order – during periods of "prohibition".[20]

3) To allow substantial comparative insights into the developments of medical plurality and medical pluralism inside the selected European countries it was necessary to limit the geographical framework of this volume. This creates a good basis for further comparisons with other parts of the world on which research has focused more intensively so far. In this volume, Manchanda already provides a glimpse on India.[21] Traditionally, the bulk of the studies on medical pluralism concern the colonies and countries of the so-called "Third World" where western biomedicine was for a long time only available to the better off.[22] Local medical traditions have for a long time played an important part in the healthcare provision of the large majority of the population and continue to do so. All sorts of hybrid forms of medicine, often including elements of biomedicine and the regional practices, have emerged as a result of colonialism and (dependant) modernization. Interaction between these various elements of knowledge and practice inside the local medical market and – to a lesser extent – the patients' choices have been considered by the anthropological and ethnographic research. Concepts of power and, more recently, subalternity have played an important role in these interactions. The research into medical pluralism in Europe might benefit more from the refined gaze on interactions between the provider and the ill person developed in the medical ethnography of the "Third World". These cultural aspects remain crucial even if they do not contribute much to a definition of medical pluralism from the historical perspective.

Bibliography

Bothe, Detlev: Neue deutsche Heilkunde 1933–1945: dargestellt anhand der Zeitschrift "Hippokrates" und der Entwicklung der volksheilkundlichen Laienbewegung. Husum 1991.
Brade, Anna-Elisabeth: Die Welt der Medizin und die Haltung der Legislative: Dänemark. In: Dinges, Martin (ed.): Weltgeschichte der Homöopathie. Länder – Schulen – Heilkundige. München 1996, pp. 132–154.
Capra, Fritjof: Wendezeit: Bausteine für ein neues Weltbild (The turning point). Bern 1983.

19 Jütte/Eklöf et al. (2001); Brade (1996); Eklöf (2008).
20 Brade (1996), p. 145. Cf. Bauberot in this volume for products of Kneipp in France.
21 Dinges: Medical Pluralism (2013).
22 Dinges (2011).

Cook, Harold John: Matters of exchange: commerce, medicine, and science in the Dutch Golden Age. New Haven 2007.

Dinges, Martin (ed.): Medizinkritische Bewegungen im Deutschen Reich (ca. 1870 – ca. 1933). Stuttgart 1996.

Dinges, Martin: Patientenpräferenzen und die öffentliche Gesundheitsversorgung in Indien. Der Versorgungsbeitrag der Homöopathie (Zweiter Teil). In: Zeitschrift für Klassische Homöopathie 55 (2011), no. 3, pp. 122–133.

Dinges, Martin: Entwicklungen der Homöopathie seit 30 Jahren. In: Zeitschrift für Klassische Homöopathie 56 (2012), no. 3, pp. 137–148.

Dinges, Martin: Aufstieg und Fall des "Halbgottes in Weiß"? Gesellschaftliches Ansehen und Selbstverständnis von Ärzten (1800–2010). In: Medizin, Gesellschaft und Geschichte 31 (2013), pp. 145–162.

Dinges, Martin (ed.): Medical Pluralism and Homeopathy in India and Germany (1810–2010). A Comparison of Practices. Stuttgart 2013.

Eklöf, Motzi: The homeopathic hospital that never was: attempts in the Swedish Riksdag (1853 to 1863) to establish a homeopathic hospital and the issue of theory versus empiricism in medicine. In: Medizin, Gesellschaft und Geschichte 26 (2008), pp. 167–206.

Flügge, Sibylla: Hebammen und heilkundige Frauen. Recht und Rechtswirklichkeit im 15. und 16. Jahrhundert. Frankfurt/Main 1998.

Haug, Alfred: Die Reichsarbeitsgemeinschaft für eine Neue Deutsche Heilkunde (1935/36): ein Beitrag zum Verhältnis von Schulmedizin, Naturheilkunde und Nationalsozialismus. Husum 1985.

Haug, Roswitha: Die Auswirkungen der NS-Doktrin auf Homöopathie und Phytotherapie: eine vergleichende Analyse von einer medizinischen und zwei pharmazeutischen Zeitschriften. Stuttgart 2009.

Illich, Ivan: Die Nemesis der Medizin: von den Grenzen des Gesundheitswesens (Limits to Medicine). Reinbek 1977.

Jankrift, Kay Peter: Krankheit und Heilkunde im Mittelalter. Darmstadt 2003.

Jütte, Robert: The Paradox of Professionalization: homeopathy and hydropathy as unorthodoxy in Germany in the 19th and 20th century. In: Jütte, Robert; Risse, Günter B.; Woodward, John (eds.): Culture, Knowledge, and Healing: Historical Perspectives of Homeopathic Medicine in Europe and North America. Sheffield 1998, pp. 65–88.

Jütte, Robert; Eklöf, Motzi et al. (eds.): Historical aspects of unconventional medicine: approaches, concepts, case studies. Sheffield 2001.

Kooreman, Peter; Baars, Erik: Patients whose GP knows complementary medicine tend to have lower costs and live longer. In: The European Journal of Health Economics 13 (2012), no. 6, pp. 769–776.

Mildenberger, Florian: Medikale Subkulturen in der Bundesrepublik Deutschland und ihre Gegner (1950–1990): die Zentrale zur Bekämpfung der Unlauterkeit im Heilgewerbe. Stuttgart 2011.

Schlumbohm, Jürgen: Lebendige Phantome. Ein Entbindungshospital und seine Patienten 1751–1830. Göttingen 2012.

Seidel, Hans-Christoph: Eine neue "Kultur des Gebärens": die Medikalisierung von Geburt im 18. und 19. Jahrhundert in Deutschland. Stuttgart 1998.

Stein, Claudia: Die Behandlung der Franzosenkrankheit in der Frühen Neuzeit am Beispiel Augsburgs. Stuttgart 2003.

Studer, Hans Peter; Busato, André: Ist ärztliche Komplementärmedizin wirtschaftlich? In: Schweizerische Ärztezeitung 91 (2010), no. 18, pp. 707–711.

Walach, Harald; Weidenhammer, Wolfgang (eds.): Insights into the Current Situation of CAM in Europe: Major Findings of the EU Project CAMbrella. (=Forschende Komplementärmedizin 19 (2012), Suppl. 2) Freiburg/Brsg. 2012.

MEDIZIN, GESELLSCHAFT UND GESCHICHTE — BEIHEFTE

Herausgegeben von Robert Jütte.

Franz Steiner Verlag   ISSN 0941-5033

Heil und Heilung
Geschichte der Laienheilkundigen und
Struktur antimodernistischer Welt-
anschauungen in Kaiserreich und
Weimarer Republik am Beispiel von Eugen
Wenz (1856–1945)
2000. 458 S., kt.
ISBN 978-3-515-07390-5

16. Karin Stukenbrock
„Der zerstückte Cörper"
Zur Sozialgeschichte der anatomischen
Sektionen in der frühen Neuzeit (1650–
1800)
2001. 309 S., kt.
ISBN 978-3-515-07734-0

17. Gunnar Stollberg / Ingo Tamm
**Die Binnendifferenzierung
in deutschen Krankenhäusern
bis zum Ersten Weltkrieg**
2001. 624 S. mit 4 Abb., kt.
ISBN 978-3-515-07733-0

18. Jens-Uwe Teichler
**„Der Charlatan strebt nicht
nach Wahrheit, er verlangt nur
nach Geld"**
Zur Auseinandersetzung zwischen natur-
wissenschaftlicher Medizin und Laienme-
dizin im deutschen Kaiserreich am Beispiel
von Hypnotismus und Heilmagnetismus
2002. 233 S. mit 16 Abb., kt.
ISBN 978-3-515-07976-1

19. Claudia Stein
**Die Behandlung der Franzosen-
krankheit in der Frühen Neuzeit
am Beispiel Augsburgs**
2003. 293 S., kt.
ISBN 978-3-515-08032-3

20. Jörg Melzer
Vollwerternährung
Diätetik, Naturheilkunde,
Nationalsozialismus, sozialer Anspruch
2003. 480 S., kt.
ISBN 978-3-515-08278-5

21. Thomas Gerst
**Ärztliche Standesorganisation
und Standespolitik in Deutschland
1945–1955**
2004. 270 S., kt.
ISBN 978-3-515-08056-9

22. Florian Steger
Asklepiosmedizin
Medizinischer Alltag in der römischen
Kaiserzeit
2004. 244 S. und 12 Taf. mit 17 Abb., kt.
ISBN 978-3-515-08415-4

23. Ulrike Thoms
**Anstaltskost im
Rationalisierungsprozeß**
Die Ernährung in Krankenhäusern und
Gefängnissen im 18. und 19. Jahrhundert
2005. 957 S. mit 84 Abb., kt.
ISBN 978-3-515-07935-8

24. Simone Moses
Alt und krank
Ältere Patienten in der Medizinischen
Klinik der Universität Tübingen zur Zeit
der Entstehung der Geriatrie 1880 bis 1914
2005. 277 S. mit 61 Tab. und 27 Diagr.
ISBN 978-3-515-08654-7

25. Sylvelyn Hähner-Rombach (Hg.)
„Ohne Wasser ist kein Heil"
Medizinische und kulturelle Aspekte
der Nutzung von Wasser
2005. 167 S., kt.
ISBN 978-3-515-08785-8

26. Heiner Fangerau / Karen Nolte (Hg.)
**„Moderne" Anstaltspsychiatrie
im 19. und 20. Jahrhundert**
Legitimation und Kritik
2006. 416 S., kt.
ISBN 978-3-515-08805-3

27. Martin Dinges (Hg.)
**Männlichkeit und Gesundheit
im historischen Wandel ca. 1800 –
ca. 2000**
2007. 398 S. mit 7 Abb., 22 Tab.
und 4 Diagr., kt.
ISBN 978-3-515-08920-3

28. Marion Maria Ruisinger
Patientenwege
Die Konsiliarkorrespondenz Lorenz
Heisters (1683–1758) in der Trew-
Sammlung Erlangen
2008. 308 S. mit 7 Abb. und 16 Diagr., kt.
ISBN 978-3-515-08806-0

29. Martin Dinges (Hg.)
**Krankheit in Briefen im deutschen
und französischen Sprachraum**
17.–21. Jahrhundert
2007. 267 S., kt.
ISBN 978-3-515-08949-4

30. Helen Bömelburg
Der Arzt und sein Modell
Porträtfotografien aus der deutschen Psy-
chiatrie 1880 bis 1933
2007. 239 S. mit 68 Abb. und 2 Diagr., kt.
ISBN 978-3-515-09096-8

31. Martin Krieger
Arme und Ärzte, Kranke und Kassen
Ländliche Gesundheitsversorgung und

kranke Arme in der südlichen Rheinprovinz
(1869 bis 1930)
2009. 452 S. mit 7 Abb., 16 Tab. und 5
Ktn., kt.
ISBN 978-3-515-09171-8

32. Sylvelyn Hähner-Rombach
Alltag in der Krankenpflege /
Everyday Nursing Life
Geschichte und Gegenwart /
Past and Present
2009. 309 S. mit 22 Tab., kt.
ISBN 978-3-515-09332-3

33. Nicole Schweig
Gesundheitsverhalten von Männern
Gesundheit und Krankheit in Briefen,
1800–1950
2009. 288 S. mit 4 Abb. und 8 Tab., kt.
ISBN 978-3-515-09362-0

34. Andreas Renner
Russische Autokratie
und europäische Medizin
Organisierter Wissenstransfer
im 18. Jahrhundert
2010. 373 S., kt.
ISBN 978-3-515-09640-9

35. Philipp Osten (Hg.)
Patientendokumente
Krankheit in Selbstzeugnissen
2010. 253 S. mit 3 Abb., kt.
ISBN 978-3-515-09717-8

36. Susanne Hoffmann
Gesunder Alltag im
20. Jahrhundert?
Geschlechterspezifische Diskurse und
gesundheitsrelevante Verhaltensstile
in deutschsprachigen Ländern
2010. 538 S. mit 7 Abb., kt.
ISBN 978-3-515-09681-2

37. Marion Baschin
Wer lässt sich von einem
Homöopathen behandeln?
Die Patienten des Clemens Maria Franz von
Bönninghausen (1785–1864)
2010. 495 S. mit 45 Abb., kt.
ISBN 978-3-515-09772-7

38. Ulrike Gaida
Bildungskonzepte der
Krankenpflege in der
Weimarer Republik
Die Schwesternschaft des Evangelischen

Diakonievereins e.V. Berlin-Zehlendorf
2011. 346 S. mit 12 Abb., kt.
ISBN 978-3-515-09783-3

39. Martin Dinges / Robert Jütte (ed.)
The transmission of health
practices (c. 1500 to 2000)
2011. 190 S. mit 4 Abb. und 1 Tab., kt.
ISBN 978-3-515-09897-7

40. Sylvelyn Hähner-Rombach
Gesundheit und Krankheit im
Spiegel von Petitionen an den
Landtag von Baden-Württemberg
1946 bis 1980
2011. 193 S. mit 27 Tab., kt.
ISBN 978-3-515-09914-1

41. Florian Mildenberger
Medikale Subkulturen in der
Bundesrepublik Deutschland
und ihre Gegner (1950–1990)
Die Zentrale zur Bekämpfung der
Unlauterkeit im Heilgewerbe
2011. 188 S. mit 15 Abb., kt.
ISBN 978-3-515-10041-0

42. Angela Schattner
Zwischen Familie, Heilern
und Fürsorge
Das Bewältigungsverhalten von
Epileptikern in deutschsprachigen
Gebieten des 16.–18. Jahrhunderts
2012. 299 S. mit 5 Abb. und 2 Tab., kt.
ISBN 978-3-515-09947-9

43. Susanne Rueß / Astrid Stölzle (Hg.)
Das Tagebuch der jüdischen Kriegs-
krankenschwester Rosa Bendit,
1914 bis 1917
2012. 175 S. mit 6 Abb., kt.
ISBN 978-3-515-10124-0

44. Sabine Herrmann
Giacomo Casanova und die Medizin
des 18. Jahrhunderts
2012. 214 S. mit 8 Abb., kt.
ISBN 978-3-515-10175-2

45. Florian Mildenberger
Medizinische Belehrung
für das Bürgertum
Medikale Kulturen in der Zeitschrift
„Die Gartenlaube" (1853–1944)
2012. 230 S. mit 11 Abb., kt.
ISBN 978-3-515-10232-2